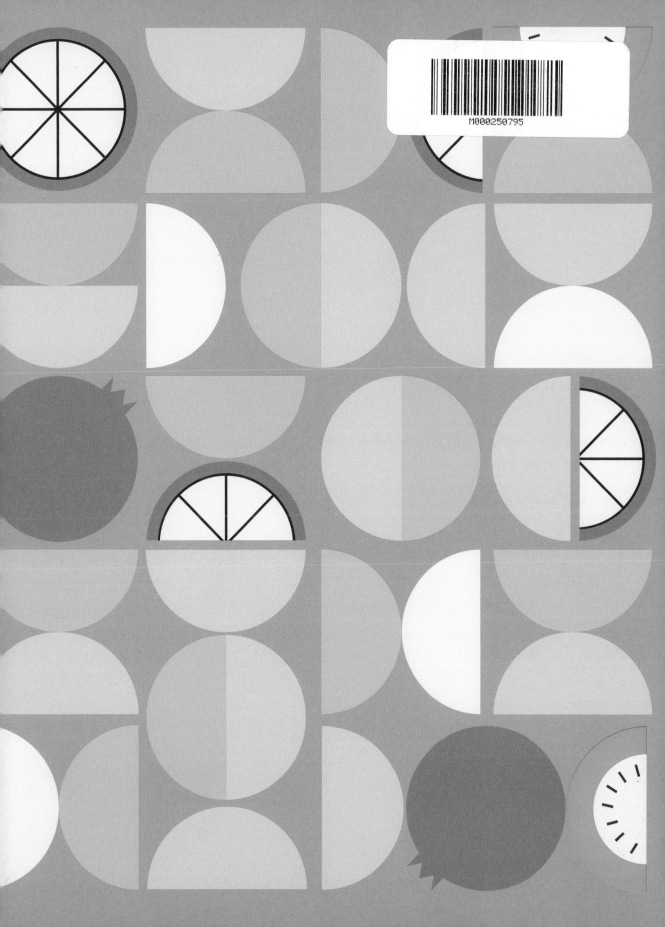

The Kitchen Prescription

Dr Saliha Mahmood Ahmed
GASTROENTEROLOGIST AND MASTERCHEF WINNER

For my baby Haadi Ahmed as he finds his own voice

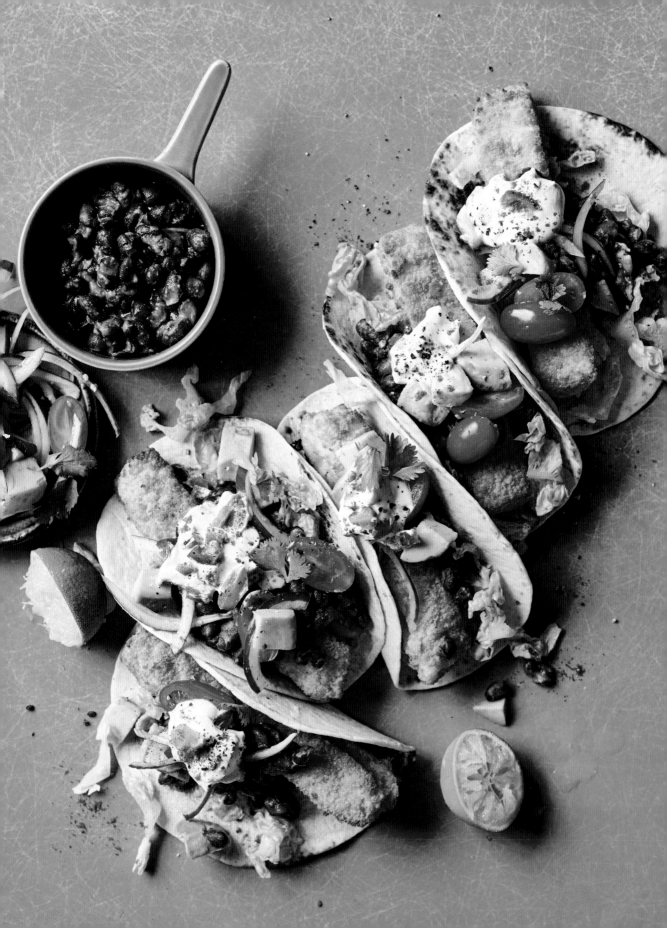

101 delicious everyday recipes to revolutionise your gut health

The Kitchen Prescription

Dr Saliha Mahmood Ahmed

GASTROENTEROLOGIST AND MASTERCHEF WINNER

Photography by Steve Joyce

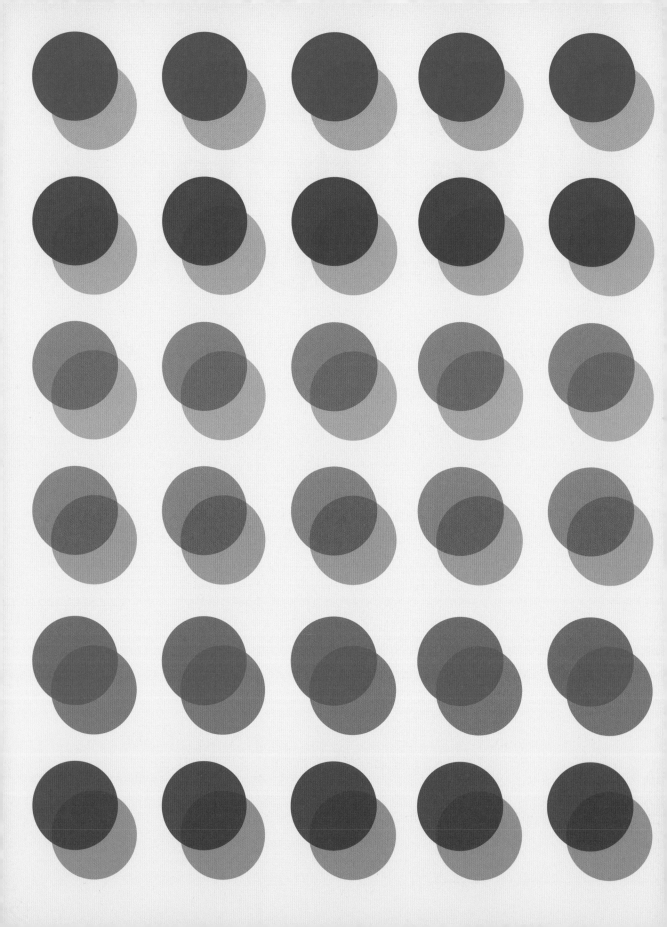

Contents

Winning *MasterChef* was undoubtedly
a turning point in my career.

In spring 2017 when the *MasterChef* final
aired, I made the dramatic transition from
junior doctor – who was also an enthusiastic
home cook and mother – to chef. Moments
after winning the competition people
started asking me whether I would quit
practising medicine and concentrate solely
on a new-found food career. My answer
back then remains the same now: food
and medicine are inexorably linked to one
another and it is an honour to be a doctor
who specialises in digestive health and can
both cook and teach others to cook.

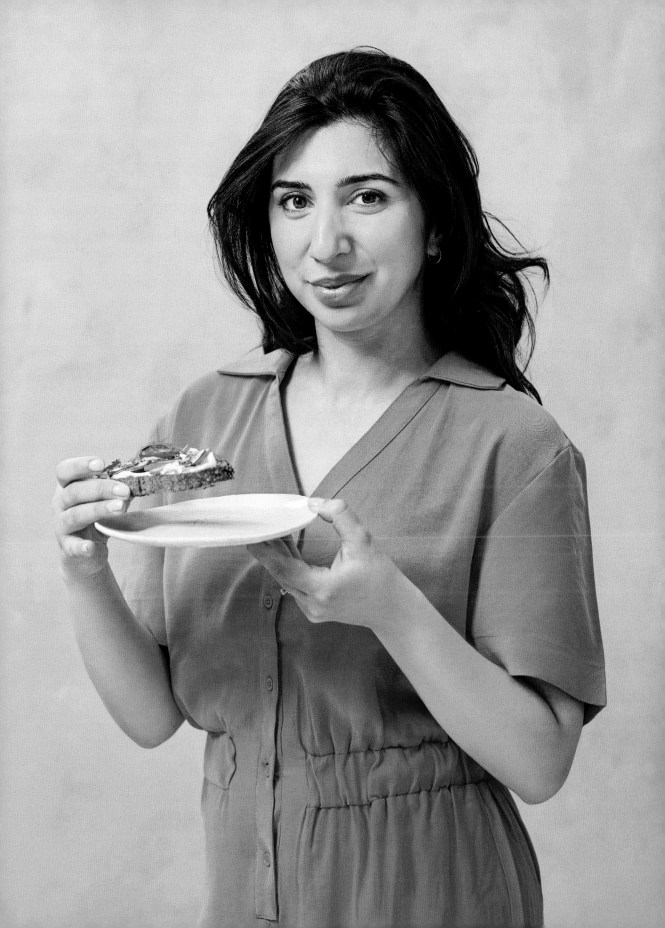

Introduction

I strongly feel that people do not realise that what they choose to eat is the single most important factor affecting their long-term health. I have been a National Health Service doctor for over a decade now and in my role as a Specialist Registrar in Gastroenterology working on the frontline, I have seen all too often the far-reaching health consequences of a poor diet. From obesity to type 2 diabetes, heart disease and many other conditions, the mortality and morbidity incurred because of a lifetime of 'unhealthy' eating patterns is utterly astounding.

Like millions of other doctors across the globe, I find myself prescribing a plethora of medications to treat an array of conditions that are fundamentally a direct consequence of poor nutrition. Although there is clearly a role for medications (and I am by no means suggesting that you stop taking them), the reality is that very few medications cure; some medications prevent decline, while others just ease suffering and control symptoms. Sometimes I see medications work wonders, many other times they just do not suffice.

When I stop looking at patients through the microscope lens of a doctor who prescribes pills and instead look at the bigger human context to evaluate the factors that led to an individual becoming my patient in the first place, there is always one key question that springs to mind: how could we have PREVENTED this person getting to the point in their illness that they find themselves in today?

Medication is invariably not the answer and, sadly, the biggest misconception of all is that you can prevent or cure all ill health with the contents of a pharmacist's cupboard. The answer does, however, lie in what an individual chooses to put on their plate, not just over a week, month or year, but over the course of a lifetime. The potential to influence people's eating habits and so help to prevent long-term disease was my motivation to write this book.

The Kitchen Prescription functions as much more than a generic 'healthy eating' cookbook. It is specifically a manual on how you can cook your way to a healthier gut. The recipes are based on the most up-to-date and robust research in an evolving scientific discipline. After reading this book you will understand how a healthier gut leads in turn to a healthier body and mind, and how if you look after your gut, your gut will look after you.

I feel the same sense of pride offering you this cookbook – with recipes designed to transform your gut health – that a laboratory scientist may feel when they discover a new medication. Food is wonderful, joyous and sensory, an emotion and sustenance all in one. That is why it brings me endless pleasure to prescribe you these joyous recipes rather than a packet of pills.

The premise of this book is that you do not have to deprive yourself, diet or go hungry. It is about improving your gut health with a diverse diet, eating delicious food cooked by a doctor-come-food-fanatic-turned-MasterChef-winner, while learning the key scientific principles of gut-healthy eating.

Through the featured recipes I hope to celebrate the joy that food brings to our lives, while also addressing the pervasive pseudo-science that surrounds the field of gut-healthy nutrition. We do exist in a bizarre food climate. There is just such a vast array of food options and lifestyle choices to choose from. Just try typing #healthyfood or #guthealth into Instagram and look at the sheer array of different options that come up . . . totally mind-boggling. How does one step away from this maelstrom of confusion?

I have found that the way to empower individuals to lead a healthy lifestyle is to firstly ask them to forget everything they know – or think they know – about healthy eating. Approach your diet as if it were a blank canvas and start from the first principles. A few key foundational concepts are fundamental, upon which the rest of our understanding of gut-healthy eating can be based. These include having an understanding of the following: what the gut microbiome is; what nutrition and digestion are; and what makes taste, well 'taste'.

After spending some time addressing these foundational concepts and before we dive straight into the recipes (if you can resist doing that), I will introduce my three-pillar prescription for how you can revolutionise your gut health and learn to eat to beat illness – from the inside out. I think of this three-pillar prescription as my three commandments of good gut health. They are as follows and will be discussed in detail going forward.

+	PRESCRIPTION 1:	COOK, COOK, COOK
+	PRESCRIPTION 2:	FEED YOUR GUT BUGS
+	PRESCRIPTION 3:	DO NOT DIET

Once you have read the foundational concepts of nutrition and the three-pillar prescription for glorious gut health, you will approach the recipes in this book with new-found scientific knowledge. Not only are the recipes simple, nutritious, family-friendly and delicious, but they are also living examples of evidence-based science in practice. By the end of the book you'll be able to cook your way to a healthy gut, with all the benefits for your overall health, without even knowing you're doing it. Magically, all you will know you are doing is eating utterly delicious food.

You will notice that unlike other books in this genre, this book won't give you nutritional breakdowns, or calorie counts; I find these old-fashioned and counterproductive for the most part. *The Kitchen Prescription* will, however, help you rethink your relationship with food so that you are better able to cater to your unique nutritional needs throughout your life, while celebrating the immense joy food brings to our lives, without a calorie count in sight.

You will however find vegetarian (V), vegan (VG) and gluten-free (GF) tags on the recipes. I'm always surprised by how many manufactured foods have gluten listed on the labels – even things like stock cubes, miso and soy sauce. Likewise for items like dark chcolate not always being vegan. It's worth always double checking the labels of the products you buy.

I have been intentionally cautious to not overstate any gut health claims. As a doctor I feel I have a great responsibility to not present conflated information; where the science is grey, I hope to present it to you as such. As scientists we must acknowledge that there are still gaps in our knowledge of what constitutes optimal gut-healthy eating. Sadly, there are no single superfoods that can change one's gut health, there is no one recipe that will cure your digestive ailments immediately. Good gut-healthy nutrition does not come in the form of a magic bullet.

However, by the end of this book you will have the tools to understand what gut-healthy eating should look like, and with it a fantastic set of recipes to draw 'gut-licious' inspiration from. I view these recipes as a starting point in your journey; they are your launch pad to springboard you into a lifetime of gut-healthy eating. Many a delicious, gut-loving meal awaits.

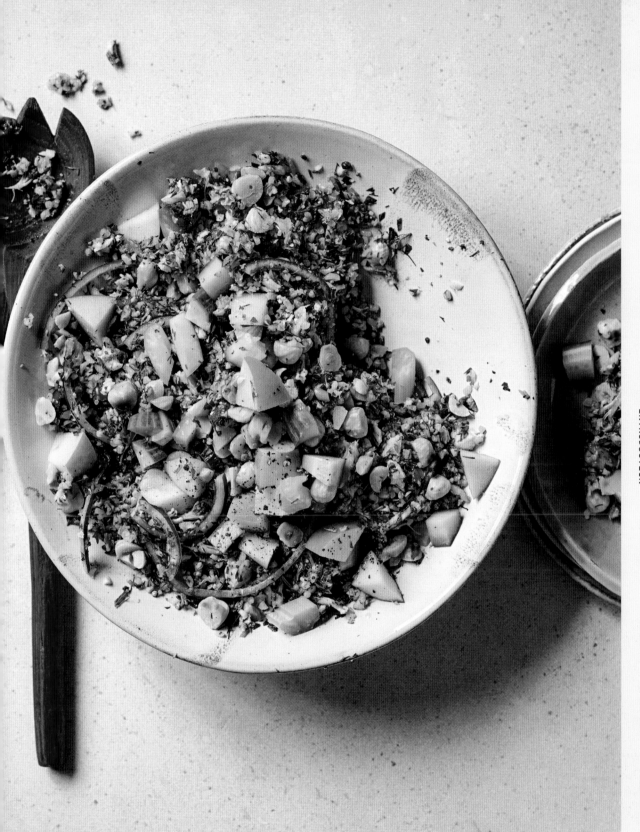

What is the gut microbiome? *

How many microbes do you think
live in your gut right now?

A million? Ten million?

As an estimate, the human gut hosts around 100 trillion (or more) microbes. For anyone who needs to conceptualise that number it is one followed by fourteen zeroes; more stars than in the entire Milky Way, more fish than in all the oceans on Earth. This gut community, called the microbiota, started to develop inside each of us after we passed through our mother's vaginal canal at birth.

Each one of these microbes possesses its own individual DNA, and the collection of genes inside all those bugs put together is called the 'microbiome'. Our gut microbiome contains literally millions of genes, and far outnumbers the 23,000 or so actual human genes inside your body. These genes produce literally thousands of metabolites and can consequently influence our fitness and health.

Every individual's gut microbiota is unique, like a personal fingerprint, and susceptible to rapid and frequent changes. This is a good thing, because if we start eating a gut-healthy diet full of different plant species (fruits, vegetables, whole grains, nuts and seeds, legumes and pulses) as reflected in the recipes in this book, we observe beneficial changes in the composition of the gut microbes fairly rapidly. If done consistently, we are talking days and short weeks – rather than months and years – for meaningful microbiome changes to be observed.

When undigested food or fibre reaches the colon, it is our microbiota that get to work, fermenting the non-digestible bits so that the body can extract even more energy from our food, energy that could not otherwise have been harvested by the small bowel. It also recycles nitrogen, sugars and fats that escaped digestion in the small bowel, and even helps with the production of vitamins B and K. But the role of our gut microbes in relation to our overall health is not limited to digestion; the microbes of the large bowel have been shown to influence the strength of our immune system, to affect our bodies' ability to keep inflammation contained, to stimulate the local nervous system, and to increase cell regeneration on the lining of the gut wall.

Scientists and nutrition experts are now in general agreement that the benefits of fostering good gut health and keeping your microbiome in tip-top shape are not restricted to the bowel. We now understand that the gut communicates with the rest of our body through the nervous system, the endocrine (hormone) system and our immune system, which means that taking care of our gut through healthy eating has an impact on virtually every cell and system in our body.

Because of these links, good gut health can allow us to reap innumerable benefits, from preventing type 2 diabetes, heart disease and stroke, to positively impacting mood and lifting clouds of depression, to a heightened sense of mental clarity and alertness – and even fighting COVID-19 infection.

Our gut microbiome has evolved with us over millions of years of human evolution and is now an essential part of our digestive process. To simplify, three main categories of 'good' bacteria exist in our guts: Bacteroidetes, Firmicutes and Prevotella actinobacteria. Each individual's gut contains different strains of these three groups in different ratios, as well as a range of other bacteria, fungi and viruses. You can even get your stool tested to see how diverse your gut microbes are. As a general rule, the more diverse your microbiome is on a scale called the Simpson's Diversity Index, the better. Astoundingly, when compared with healthy controls, lower bacterial diversity has been reproducibly observed in people suffering with inflammatory bowel disease, type 1 and type 2 diabetes, atopic eczema, coeliac disease and obesity.

Research using the most cutting-edge metagenomics sequencing techniques has identified 15 'good' gut microbes that are linked to indicators of good health, and 15 'bad' gut microbes that are strongly linked to markers of worse health (the PREDICT study). For example, Flavonifractor plautii is considered a naughty microbe, associated with less healthy foods and markers of poor health, including excess belly fat. Whereas Prevotella copri and Blastocystis are associated with steady, controlled blood sugar levels after eating.

With this new-found knowledge what is apparent is that we cannot blame one microbe for poor health and credit another for good health; it is all about the bigger picture and achieving a positive microbial balance. Each individual's microbiome is unique and their nutritional requirements are therefore also unique. There is no one-size-fits-all when it comes to dietary advice because no two people will ever have the same bugs living in their gut. The future is likely to see the development of a far more personalised approach to nutrition, whereby your optimal diet is tailored to your own gut microbiota. Sadly, we are some way away from seeing personalised nutrition rolled out into clinical practice.

The positive health consequences of having a diverse gut microbiome are completely mind-blowing. To think that it all starts with those bugs in your belly! Not a month goes by without the publication of a new high-profile scientific paper, further highlighting the beneficial impact of a diverse, healthy gut microbiome on some aspect of health. Although we are discovering more every day, it is clear that a healthy gut microbiome will lead to a healthy body and mind, so it is well worth caring for it.

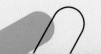

What is nutrition?

Nutrition is a fundamental part of living; it is present from cradle to grave and has a role in fuelling all life processes. Sadly, many doctors do not give the science of nutrition the due credence it deserves, a point of great contention for me. I believe that nutrition is the very foundation of preventative medicine, the cornerstone of curative medicine and the fundamental responsibility of every physician.

If you are an obstetrician, you will be concerned with the nutrition of the foetus, as well as the management of the mother's anaemia. As a paediatrician, balanced nutrition is vital, as without it our children are unable to achieve normal growth and development and reach their full potential. As a hospital medic, I know how essential nutrition is in managing diabetics, hypertension, heart disease, liver disease, the malnourished and more. As a geriatrician you may observe that the outcomes of good and bad eating patterns are all the more evident in the latter years of one's life. As doctors, we should not just be treating disease, but treating the individual who has the disease. By addressing poor nutrition in our patients, we can make an immense difference to their long-term quality of life.

Well-nourished people have the best chance of fighting disease and this nourishment comes in the form of macronutrients, which are the dietary big guns (carbohydrate, protein and fat) that are vital sources of energy and which we need in relatively large amounts, and micronutrients (various vitamins and minerals), which are vital for many bodily functions, but needed in much smaller amounts. The gut-healthy recipes featured in this book are designed to showcase an array of delightful macro- and micronutrients.

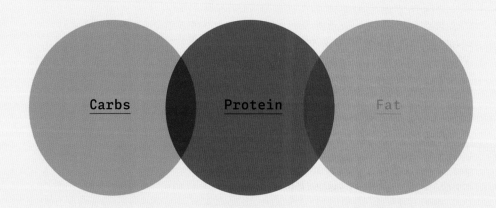

Carbs   Protein   Fat

Macronutrients

+ Carbohydrates:

What would life be without a bowl of pasta? We need carbohydrates to sustain life, to fuel our tissues, to pump blood through our beating heart, even to power the brain and make us the sentient, thinking being we are. Think back to the last time you avoided carbohydrates, either intentionally or unintentionally. Did it affect your concentration and energy levels? I bet it did. So, what are they?

Carbohydrates can be either simple or complex. Simple carbohydrates are made up of either one or two sugar molecules bonded together e.g. glucose and fructose in fruit and honey, galactose and lactose in dairy products, sucrose in sugar cane or maltose in molasses. On the other hand, complex carbohydrates (otherwise known as starches) are made of hundreds and thousands of monosaccharide units all joined together. These are the carbohydrates you find in beans and whole grains. Fibre is any complex carbohydrate that cannot be broken down in the small bowel and therefore moves down whole in its unmodified state into the colon, where it is the perfect food for our gut bugs.

Lots of people talk about whether carbohydrates are 'good' or 'bad' for us. This is not a helpful distinction since all foods have their place in our diet and we have to find a balance that works for us as individuals. In fact, you will notice an array of recipes in this book that feature carbohydrates, from **Sunshine Tomatoes and Labneh on Toast (page 62)** to **Spiced Potato Salad with Tomatoes and Broad Beans (page 81)**, **Chipotle Chilli Wild Rice (page 94)**, **Broccoli Spaghetti with Herby Chermoula (page 180)**, **Kimchi and Garlic Fried Rice (page 160)** and more. *The Kitchen Prescription* is in no way founded on the carbohydrate restricting 'keto diet' principle – which will be some consolation for the spud, rice, toast and pasta lovers among us.

Having said that, it is important to recognise that not all carbohydrates are created equal. The carbohydrates that you get in their natural, nutrient-dense form, for example in whole grains, quinoa, vegetables, barley, oats and beans, are rich in fibre and more nutritious and gut-healthy than the refined carbohydrates found in white bread, or the croissant you have with your cup of coffee.

Excess amounts of refined carbohydrates are also linked with weight gain and metabolic diseases. It is not so much about whether you eat carbohydrates or not, rather which carbohydrates you choose to eat. Around one third of your daily intake should come from carbohydrates, so it is well worth making sure you know which carbohydrates your food contains.

The trick is to consume fewer refined carbohydrates and more complex carbohydrates where possible. Complex carbs resist early digestion in the small bowel and so enter the large bowel, where microbes can then feed on these gut-healthy complex carbohydrates. To get more complex carbs into your diet try bulgur wheat, pearl barley, wild rice, quinoa, rye bread and sourdough. With time you can even start getting experimental with your carbohydrates, enjoying varieties like freekeh and sorghum.

+ Protein:

Our bone, muscles, skin, blood, hair and nails – in fact ALL of our bodies' cells – contain protein. In fact, after water, protein is the second most abundant compound in the human body.

There are 20 amino acids in total that make protein in our bodies. Of those 20 amino acids, all but nine can be made by the body. Those nine amino acids that our bodies can't synthesise are called 'essential' amino acids.

If a particular food contains all nine essential amino acids, it is called a 'complete' protein. Examples include milk, eggs, yoghurt, fish and meat. Plant-based sources of complete proteins are quinoa, soya and hemp. Sources of 'incomplete' proteins (foods that contain fewer than the nine essential amino acids) include legumes, pulses, grains, nuts, seeds and many vegetables.

However, these terms can be misleading. The terms 'complete' and 'incomplete' only reflect the ability of one food to meet all essential amino acid needs, as opposed to considering whether you have met your essential amino acid requirement through the various foods you have eaten through the course of the day. So, rest assured, incomplete proteins are still a vital and healthy part of your diet.

The recipes in *The Kitchen Prescription* are abundant in essential amino acids and eating a variety of them will ensure that you get enough protein to build body tissues, whether that is in the form of a mouth-watering **Berbere Chicken (page 220)** or a **Chickpea, Fenugreek and Okra Curry (page 138)**.

The amount of protein we need varies across the course of our lives; it changes during pregnancy and lactation, and as we grow older our requirement increases. For those people who take part in very vigorous physical activity, some protein after training sessions can help to rebuild muscles. As a rough guide for those who like counting (not me), the recommended protein intake is approximately 56g a day for men and approximately 45g a day for women (depending on body weight).

For those of us who are not bodybuilders, the most important consideration is not how much protein we are getting but where we are getting that protein from. I am not vegan or vegetarian, but you will notice that the majority of the recipes I have included in this book are plant-based. This is intentional. It is my belief that too much of our protein comes from red or processed meat and that we need to shift this balance back towards plant sources. You will notice that I use no processed meats at all in the recipes and less than a handful of recipes feature red meat. There is some fish and chicken across the chapters, but most lunch and dinner recipes are devised to be vegetarian or vegan. Eating more nuts, legumes or pulses, for instance, or going 'meat free' for a few days a week won't affect your protein status, nor will swapping tofu for chicken in your stir-fry, or choosing a bean burger over a beef burger every so often. What it will do is improve the variety of proteins that your body is able to access, along with all the other goodness that is present in those non-meat sources of protein.

And if you are vegan, rest assured that provided you eat a varied diet, you will get plenty of the various essential amino acids you need from the different foods you eat across the course of the day or week.

Try this useful exercise: reflect back on the meals that you have eaten for dinner in the preceding week. How many of them featured meat as the main source of protein? If you find that the majority of your dinners last week were indeed animal protein-based, then this is something that you can address using inspiration from the recipes featured in this book. How about swapping your regular cottage pie for a lentil-based **Gut-healing Masala Cottage Pie (page 182)**, switching your traditional meat lasagne to a lighter, brighter, gut-friendly **Za'atar Lasagne Verde (page 164)** or exchanging a pepperoni pizza for home-made **Primavera Pizza (page 162)**?

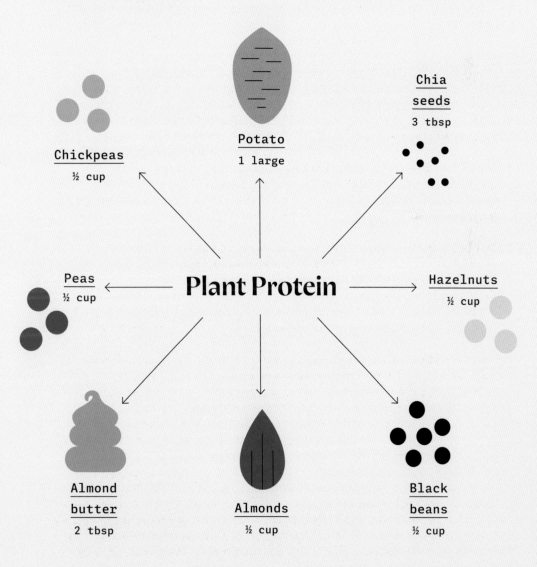

Chickpeas
½ cup

Potato
1 large

Chia
seeds
3 tbsp

Peas
½ cup

Plant Protein

Hazelnuts
½ cup

Almond
butter
2 tbsp

Almonds
½ cup

Black
beans
½ cup

+ Fat:

Fat is an incredibly important part of the diet. Instead of vilifying it and blaming it for all our food-related health issues, we need to start seeing it for the macronutrient hero it is. Fats are the most energy-dense nutrient around, but they also carry soluble vitamins like vitamins A, D, E and K around the body and help the body to utilise them.

Fats can be classified into saturated and unsaturated varieties. Saturated fats tend to be solid at room temperature and from animal sources, while unsaturated fats are usually liquid and from plant sources. Unsaturated fats can be further sub-classified into polyunsaturated or monounsaturated fats. These distinctions are important, though confusing even for me as a gastroenterologist and chef.

Although most foods contain a mixture of saturated and unsaturated fats, the dominant type is the one that we tend to stick with in our descriptions. For example, over half of butter is saturated fat and a quarter is monounsaturated, so to make things simple we describe butter as a saturated fat. As mentioned, the fats found in animal products (including cheese and cream) are all sources of saturated fats: think of the most delicious things in the world – the cakes, the potato dauphinoise, the fatty bits of a steak, a cheese and onion puff pastry. Sadly, an excessive intake of saturated fats (particularly in highly processed foods) is generally considered by nutrition experts as something to avoid, as it has been fairly conclusively linked to increases in blood cholesterol and the risk of heart disease.

Unsaturated fats, abundant in plant-based foods like seeds, nuts, olives and avocados as well as olive oil, rapeseed oil, sunflower oil, corn oil, for example, are a different kettle of fish. These fats, split into monounsaturated and polyunsaturated fats, carry out different jobs in the body. Therefore, it's always recommended to get a good amount of both types of unsaturated fat (mono and poly) into your diet, which you can easily achieve with a varied, plant-based diet.

One type of unsaturated fat, in particular, is worth a specific mention: omega-3 fatty acid. This is found in oily fish, but also flaxseed (linseed) and hemp, and is associated with reduced incidence of neurodegenerative diseases, heart disease and diabetes. Robust data suggests that higher levels of omega-3 fats in the diet lead to a more diverse microbiome. So, pretty useful then. **Mackerel Salad Sandwiches (page 84)** are a classic example of how you can utilise a lesser celebrated oily omega-3-rich fish in your culinary repertoire.

Again, the question is not whether or not fat is 'good' or 'bad', but more what type of fat you eat and from where your fats come from in your diet. The key, as reflected in the recipes in this book, is to try to replace saturated fats with unsaturated fats, wherever possible. My recipe for the **Olive, Seed and Pistachio Chermoula (page 180)** is an example of how a simple herby relish can be enriched with gut-loving unsaturated fats; it is delicious tossed into pasta or over a **Baked Sweet Potato (page 148)**.

Healthy fats

Contrary to popular belief, 'low fat' diets are not
in vogue! Research tells us that healthy fats are
in fact essential and beneficial to our health.

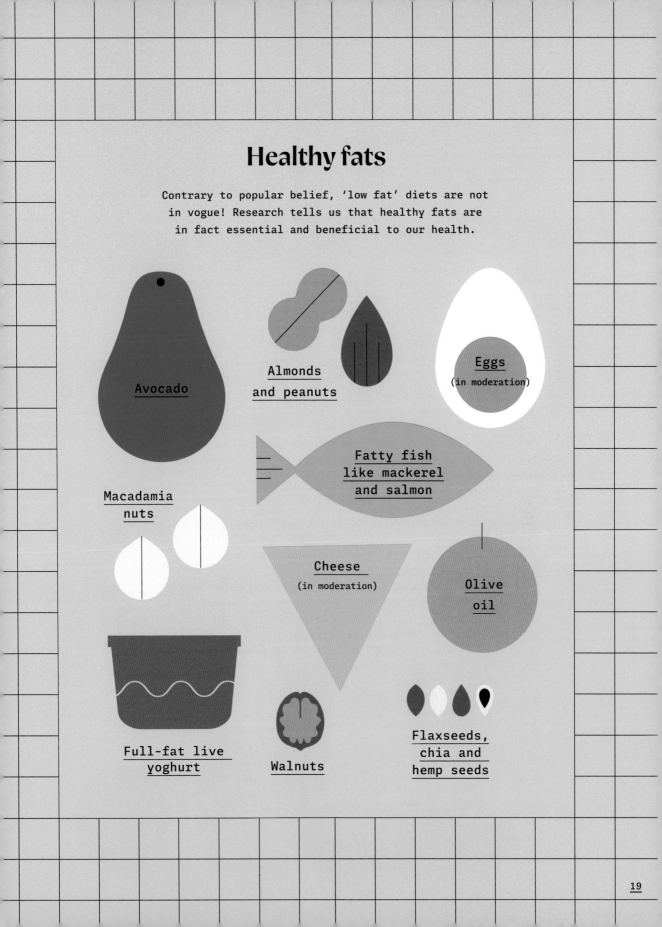

Avocado

Almonds
and peanuts

Eggs
(in moderation)

Macadamia
nuts

Fatty fish
like mackerel
and salmon

Cheese
(in moderation)

Olive
oil

Full-fat live
yoghurt

Walnuts

Flaxseeds,
chia and
hemp seeds

Micronutrients

Micronutrients are vitamins and minerals; they are the nutrients that we only need in small quantities, but the absence of which can have dramatic consequences for our health, energy levels, mental clarity and overall capacity to function.

One example that I see a lot in my clinics is iron deficiency. I have met anaemic patients who are so profoundly tired that they can't climb stairs, are breathless on minimal exertion, who suffer with excruciating chest pain and even, in extreme cases, who collapse without warning. But how much iron do we need each day to ward off these debilitating effects? It's just 8 milligrams per day (1 milligram is one thousandth of a gram) or approximately a quarter of the weight of one staple. This unnoticeable little sliver of metal can be the difference between a life free of pain and stress, and one where every day can be agony. This is the same for any of the many micronutrients we need; without 65mg of vitamin C per day we can develop scurvy where our teeth fall out; without 10mg of zinc per day, our bodies can suffer from hair loss, lack of alertness and a reduced sense of taste and smell.

With the exception of vitamin D, micronutrients are not produced by the body and have to be derived from the diet. To get those vital but imperceptible doses of micronutrients you have to opt for a colourful diet, in other words EAT THE RAINBOW. Fruit and vegetables in a range of colours, textures and flavours are nature's gift to our bellies. Just flicking through the food photographs in this book will give you a sense of the vibrancy of the multicoloured range of vitamin- and mineral-rich ingredients used across the recipes. This is something to emulate in your kitchen so don't hesitate to add colourful fruit and veg to your plate. My recipes for **Green Gut Goddess Salad (page 90)** or **Ruby Red Polyphenol Salad (page 86)** illustrate just how delicious the rainbow tastes.

I feel most people I speak to form habitual relationships with vegetables, opting for a small selection that they eat repeatedly. Once in a while buy vegetables from the supermarket that you just don't normally get. Instead of adding the usual onions, peppers and courgettes to your weekly shop, try kale, fennel and red cabbage for a change. This will allow you to eat a range of different micronutrients and your gut will thank you for the plant-based diversity it is getting – plus you will be forced to cook something new.

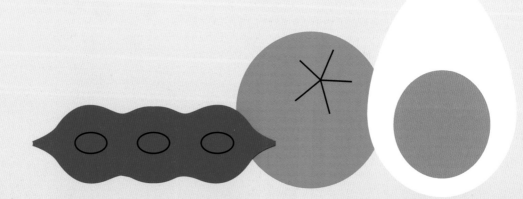

Although a complete summary of micronutrients could be the content of a separate book in itself, let's look at a few of these micronutrients in some more detail:

+

Vitamin B: There are lots of different types of vitamin B, such as thiamine, riboflavin, niacin, folate, and many others. These varieties are all water soluble and play an important role in keeping the nervous system healthy, in maintaining the eyes and skin, and in helping the body release energy from food. You can get the majority of B vitamins from foods such as peas, bananas, eggs, soya beans, edamame beans, leafy greens and chickpeas, while B12 is only found in animal products like eggs, meat, or fish. Some healthcare professionals suggest that vitamin B12 should be supplemented in vegan diets.

+

Vitamin D: This micronutrient helps us to regulate the amount of calcium and phosphate in the body, and therefore helps to keep our bones, teeth and muscles healthy. In children, vitamin D deficiency is called rickets, while in adults it is called osteomalacia. Our bodies can make vitamin D as long as we have exposure to sunlight, but in the UK some of you might have noticed that the sun sometimes doesn't make an appearance for weeks on end. This is actually a real issue; we don't get enough sun in the autumn and winter months, which puts many of us at risk of vitamin D deficiency. There is even some emerging evidence that vitamin D deficiency can exacerbate inflammatory bowel disease (Crohn's and colitis) because of its effects on local intestinal inflammation.

Sources of vitamin D include oily fish, red meat, liver and egg yolks.

+

Vitamin E: This fat-soluble vitamin comes in several forms, but the one that is used in the human body is called alpha-tocopherol. Its main role is to act as an antioxidant, a type of compound that works to prevent damage to our bodies' cells and helps them repair. It is found in almonds, pumpkins, avocados, sunflower seeds, peanuts, peppers, and many more foods. Deficiency in vitamin E can damage the back of the eyes, the nerves of the hands and feet, and can even result in impaired immune responses and a loss of control of body movements.

Vitamin K: This is another fat-soluble vitamin that comes in two forms. The main type is called phylloquinone, found in green leafy vegetables like kale, spinach, turnip greens, broccoli, Brussels sprouts and rocket – all firm favourites of mine.

The other type is called menaquinones, which are found in fermented foods like nattō as well as in small amounts in meat, cheese and eggs. Vitamin K is needed to make the various proteins required for blood clotting and the building of bones.

Iodine: This is a trace mineral that our bodies need to optimise the function of our thyroid glands, extremely important organs which control the body's metabolism. It is also needed for the development of babies' brains during pregnancy and early life.

The richest sources of iodine are fish, shellfish, dairy products like milk, and seaweed. Many of us can be iodine-deficient without realising it, but severe deficiency results in the development of goitres, another word for swelling in the neck.

Calcium: An important mineral at all ages due to its effect on bones and teeth, calcium is also needed for healthy muscle and nerve function. The requirement for calcium varies across life, particularly in breastfeeding women. We all know the foods which are rich in calcium: milk, yoghurt, cheese and other dairy products are all full of calcium. Those who cannot (or choose not to) eat dairy, for instance lactose-intolerant people or those opting for a vegan diet, can get their calcium intake from plant milks fortified with extra calcium, or calcium-fortified bread, calcium-set tofu, calcium-fortified cereal, oranges, broccoli, kale and spring greens. Spinach, dried fruits, beans, seeds and nuts also contain calcium, but they also contain compounds called oxalates or phytates, which reduce how much calcium our bodies can extract from these foods. For this reason, the British Dietetic Association recommends that we don't rely on these foods as our main sources of calcium.

Now that we have had a look at what macronutrients and micronutrients are, the next logical step is to try to understand which foods make up a gut-healthy diet. The concept of gut-healthy eating is shifting, based on evolving knowledge of the microbiome and how it is impacted by food. What we know today is not what we knew ten years ago and what we know in ten years may be different to what we know today.

Nutrition research is notoriously difficult and time-consuming, but we can, however, learn a lot from patterns of eating across different population groups. Certain societies have very specific diets and three successful dietary patterns of eating that we can learn from are the Mediterranean diet, the Nordic diet and the Japanese diet. Data gathered from years (actually decades) of observation shows that that the people who eat these diets typically live long, healthy lives. There must be a reason for this, so the question becomes: what can we learn about their secrets to success?

When you take a trip to southern Italy or Greece, the older people almost radiate health. They might look frail, or a bit wrinkled; no one is suggesting that they've discovered the elixir of eternal youth, but internally they are running like well-oiled machines with very low rates of chronic illness. They lead non-sedentary lifestyles, and the core of their diet focuses on plants – seasonal, fresh and delicious. They don't hold back on their healthy unsaturated fats; olive oil gets drizzled over virtually everything, but animal protein consumption from fish and poultry is traditionally low, as is the intake of red meat and eggs. Carbohydrates are welcomed and celebrated; think of what Italian cuisine would look like without pizza or pasta.

Similarly, the Nordic diet relies heavily on locally sourced, sustainable, plant-based meals. Sea and lake fish, lean game meats and rapeseed oil (a monounsaturated fat similar to olive oil) also feature heavily. The Nordic diet, just like the Mediterranean diet, focuses on whole foods, peas, cabbage and root vegetables; think plates of seared salmon with creamed barley and Savoy cabbage, rye bread, beetroot gravadlax, plenty of turnips and a high-protein yoghurt like Skyr to round it all off. It's enough to unleash your inner Viking.

Last, but by no means least, of our trio is the Japanese diet. The Japanese have the lowest rates of obesity and the highest life expectancies in the world, so they must be doing something very right. Okinawa, in particular, has the dual distinction of having the highest number of centenarians in the world, and also the lowest risk globally of diabetes, cancer, arthritis and Alzheimer's disease. The diet is largely fresh and unprocessed with very little in terms of refined foods or sugar. Rice, grains, vegetables like purple sweet potato, Chinese okra, bitter melon and cabbage feature heavily, as do soya beans in the form of tofu, fish and seaweed. The amount of animal products consumed is pretty moderate, and usually acts as an accompaniment to a vegetable in the dish rather than as the main attraction. Another key factor is that the Japanese are taught from childhood to eat *hara hachi bu*, or until they are 80 per cent full.

Three very different ways of eating, three diverse, rich food cultures, but one common result: healthy and long-living populations. But what is the common thread across these three diets, and what can we learn from them? Better yet, can we isolate some of the good stuff in these diets and introduce them into ours?

The common thread that I can immediately spot is that all three diets focus on consuming a wide range of different plant-based foods as the main bulk of meals, while encouraging a low level of reliance on animal-based foods, particularly red and processed meats. What's more, if you overlay the diets of these three cultures, you begin notice something rather interesting.

Successful diets are all dominated by five key plant-based food groups, shown opposite

The really good news is that our gut microbes love fruit and vegetables, whole grains, legumes, pulses, nuts and seeds too. The wider diversity of them that you eat, the more diverse your gut microbiome will become. Evidence from epidemiologic and clinical data indicates that if you include these five key food groups (fruit and veg, whole grains, legumes, pulses, and seeds and nuts) in your diet, you reduce the risk of developing a myriad of non-communicable diseases, ranging from heart disease to diabetes; there is even evidence that certain cancers could be avoided by building your diet around these five food groups. How these foods groups do this is not 100 per cent clear, but what is clear is that a large part of it is to do with the way these foods beneficially impact the gut microbiome.

The Kitchen Prescription will teach you how to seamlessly integrate these five key food groups into your daily life in a way that is as stress-free and effortless as possible. Because it is one thing knowing which foods you should be eating, and another actually knowing how to incorporate them into your diet, and yet another to be able to do so with the ingredients available from your local supermarket. By cooking the recipes in this book, you will be able to unlock the health-boosting potential of your gut microbiome, one plate of food at a time.

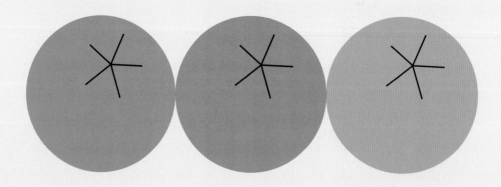

Key components of a successful diet

1

<u>Fruit and vegetables</u>
make up the bulk of
each meal; five a day
is the minimum, not
the goal.

2

<u>Whole grains</u>
are celebrated;
oats, barley, rye,
spelt, wholewheat,
brown rice, quinoa
and freekeh are
our bodies'
best friends.

3

<u>Legumes</u> such as green
beans, runner beans, and
soya beans are essential.

4

<u>Pulses</u> feature heavily
as a healthy source
of plant protein. This
includes beans, peas
and lentils.

5

<u>Seeds and nuts </u>
such as pumpkin
seeds, sunflower
seeds, sesame
seeds, peanuts,
and cashews are
popular as
snacks.

What is digestion?

You do it subconsciously all the time, but do you really understand what is going on?

In the language of science, digestion is the process of taking in food and converting it to energy for use in growth, metabolism and repair. Digestion takes place in the gut; the gut is a sophisticated piece of tubing, a bit like the engine room of the body that extends from mouth to anus.

Let's take a look at the main components of your digestive system.

+ The mouth:

The tongue tastes everything it goes past, courtesy of around 10,000 taste buds. Working with the teeth and cheeks, the tongue helps with mechanical and chemical digestion of food and creates a ball of food, which is then swallowed. Swallowing sounds simple but it is actually a complex neuromuscular process that coordinates the passage of food from the mouth to the oesophagus.

Before we swallow, we chew. The production of sufficient amounts of saliva is essential for good chewing. Some estimate that we make 20,000 litres or so in a lifetime, which would fill around a massive 60 bathtubs. Saliva starts the breakdown process of two key macronutrient groups: carbohydrates and proteins. This is due to amylase and protease enzymes, which function in a very similar way to those found in bioactive washing powders.

+ The stomach:

The widest part of the digestive tract with some serious storage capacity, a good thing when you think of the last time you were able to eat an 12-inch pizza, large chips and chicken wings all by yourself in one sitting.

The cells that line the stomach secrete incredibly powerful acids, which aid digestion and are the first line of antimicrobial defence for the body. Anyone who has suffered with acid reflux will testify just how powerful these acids are.

The stomach churns our food under subconscious control, macerating it and mixing it with a host of enzymes to form a mushy liquid called chyme. The stomach also triggers the release of an orchestra of hormones, some of which help to control our appetite, while others manage the secretions of enzymes. Luckily for us, the stomach is designed to not digest itself, as it is lined by a thick layer of mucus, which protects its rapidly regenerating lining.

Incredibly, our emotions can influence movements of the stomach. Although the extent of this varies from individual to individual, evidence suggests that sadness and fear may decrease stomach motility, while and anger and aggression may increase it. Intense pain in any part of the body will inhibit movement throughout the digestive tract, while extreme stress has been observed to have an effect on the mucus lining of the stomach too (hence why we often associate heartburn with stress).

+ The small intestine:

Also known as the small bowel, this is the main processing centre of the digestive tract. It is made up of about 6 metres or so of snake-like coiled-up tubing and is where the majority of the body's digestion and absorption of nutrients take place. It's ironic that we call it the 'small' intestine, given that it is longer than the large intestine.

The small intestine is lined with tiny hair-like projections known as villi, which under a microscope look finger-like, creating the appearance of a shag-pile rug. The villi help to maximise the surface area available in the small bowel for nutrient and water absorption; laid flat the surface of the small bowel could spectacularly almost cover a tennis court. The blood supply connected to each villi carries the absorbed nutrients away, via the liver, to the rest of the body.

+ The large intestine (colon):

The undigested contents of the small intestine enter the large intestine through a one-way valve called the ileocecal valve. From here, there's only one way out. The first part of the colon is called the caecum, which is connected to the appendix. Previously thought to be useless, we now know that the appendix acts as a reservoir for beneficial microbes, keeping the colon teeming with the living organisms that live symbiotically within the gut (more on this later). When we take antibiotics, or have a colonic, or even have a bad case of diarrhoea, this colony of microbes (called the microbiome) can be destroyed; the appendix gives us the vital seed microbes that we use to repopulate our gut.

The colon is a glorified fermentation tank, working on all the undigested bits the small bowel is unable to break down. The colon is also responsible for absorption of water, and for processing a variety of vitamins (mainly B and K) and bile salts. The colon rises up the right side of the body, across the top of the abdomen and then down the left, where it eventually transitions to the rectum and anus. The fermentation that takes place in the colon also creates a variety of gaseous by-products in the process.

What is taste?

For a sense that you have had since you were a baby, you probably don't know much about how you taste your food. The way I think about taste is that it is equal parts science and emotion; what makes this food taste the way it does? And why does it make me feel so good?

Understanding the workings of taste and the building blocks of flavour is a vital step on the journey to seeking good gut health. This is because one of the critical steps to achieving good gut health is allowing yourself to cook the most delicious, tongue-tantalising food, which excites the emotions and senses in equal measure. Gut-healthy food is not, and should not be, bland and boring; it MUST excite the taste buds.

The ability to taste has contributed a huge amount to human evolution, as it allowed early humans to know which foods were safe, which were not, which were full of calories etc. This therefore allowed them to feed their growing bodies and brains.

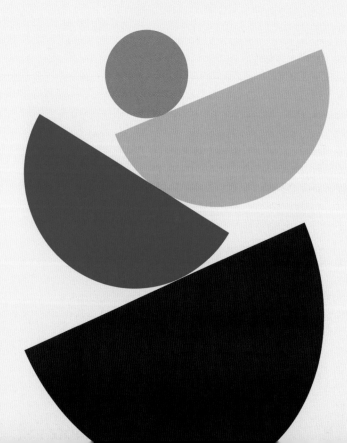

From the 4th century BC we know that humans were able to discern a selection of basic tastes as follows:

\+ **Sweet:** Creatures are evolutionarily designed to crave sweet things for sugar and calories; it's why hummingbirds search for sweet nectar to fuel their bodies, and why toddlers search for gummy bears to fuel theirs. This taste receptor, therefore, is essential to recognise food that we can derive energy from. For more on this taste see the desserts chapter (pages 228–47).

\+ **Salty:** Our bodies need salt and other minerals to function and maintain the fluid balance of our cells. Bizarrely, the specific receptor mechanisms that are involved in tasting salty food are yet to be fully understood; we know they work, but we don't quite know how.

\+ **Sour:** Scientists still aren't quite sure why we've developed taste buds for this taste since, in many ways, knowing if a food is sour doesn't tell us anything particularly useful in evolutionary terms; other flavours can, for instance, tell us if a food is going to give us energy, or if it's going to poison us. Sour foods like citrus fruits are a good source of vitamin C, but that's probably just a small part of the whole picture of why we developed the ability to taste sour.

\+ **Bitter:** A sensitivity to bitter was very handy for early humans because it was quite common for bitter foods to kill, or at least make them feel very ill. So, knowing which foods to avoid, or which foods to stop eating after taking a bite, was a very useful evolutionary skill. Modern cuisine often celebrates this divisive taste, and I find subtle bitter tastes highly complex and exciting. For example, I use the bitter notes of radicchio or dark chocolate, or the bitter bite of a grapefruit as featured in Grapefruit and Lentils with Thai-style Dressing (page 128) or Radicchio, Plum and Seared Steak Salad (page 216).

\+ **Umami:** This is the meaty savouriness that we get from condiments like Marmite, brown sauce and fish sauce, and which is also present in lamb, tomatoes, peas, asparagus, cheese, anchovies and more. Scientists have found evidence to suggest that this taste sensation is related to animals needing to be nourished with protein, as umami may be a good indicator that the food being eaten is protein-rich.

Chilli heat or 'spiciness' is not thought of as a taste. Capsaicin, the active compound in chilli, is detected by the same receptors that detect temperature in the mouth, rather than by the taste buds.

So how does taste work? Each human taste bud is a column-shaped cell, and these cells cluster to make up thousands of receptor bundles shaped like garlic bulbs. These are our taste buds; at the bottom of these bulb-like structures is a network of nerves that carry information away from the taste buds to the medulla, a primitive part of the brain that controls our basic functions.

The medulla sends taste signals onwards to an area called the insular cortex. This area of the brain is where we perceive taste, but interestingly, the insular cortex not only tells us what we are tasting, but is also one of the areas of the brain responsible for responding to visceral or emotional experiences.

The insular cortex also forwards information to the amygdala, which is responsible for the production and release of dopamine. You may have heard of this chemical before; it's the feel-good chemical that creates our sense of pleasure and reward. It's why food, especially sweet things, can be addictive; there really is a chemical reason why we go weak-kneed after taking a mouthful of chocolate fondant with its molten centre, but also why we can't stop at one.

However, the link between the insular cortex and other areas of the brain isn't limited to just the amygdala; studies in which participants ate their favourite foods under an MRI scanner showed that the experience of eating these foods also lit up other areas of the brain linked to memory, lust, love, longing, heartache, contentment and gratification, among countless others. It's why food is so enjoyable; it's not just about nutrition, it's also an experience that ignites almost every area of our brains and bodies. Taking the time to understand our personal emotional and mental connection to food is crucial if we are to succeed in revolutionising our gut health.

Taste and smell are also closely intertwined. Some scientists believe that up to 80 per cent of our experience of flavour comes from the sense of smell. This makes sense when we realise that our sense of smell outperforms virtually all our other senses when it comes to the number of different stimuli it can distinguish. Each morsel of food we eat contains millions of smell cells, known as volatile aromatic compounds. A volatile compound is essentially a chemical that moves through the air, and aromatic here refers to any chemical that the human olfactory system can register.

The volatile aromatic compounds emitted from our roast dinner are drawn to the back of the nose and throat through our breathing, and bind with a specific receptor cell which, through a complex network of nerves, fires a signal to the brain. In the brain, the aroma associated with that compound can be interpreted. When that food enters the mouth and is broken down by chewing, even more aromatic molecules burst out and hit the back of the throat and nose where they bind with other receptor cells and amplify the taste of the food we are experiencing, allowing us to experience those magical complexities of flavour. Basically, volatile compounds are the bridge between our sense of taste and smell and are what create the flavour profiles that we recognise, such as fruity, floral, citrusy, herbal, earthy or meaty.

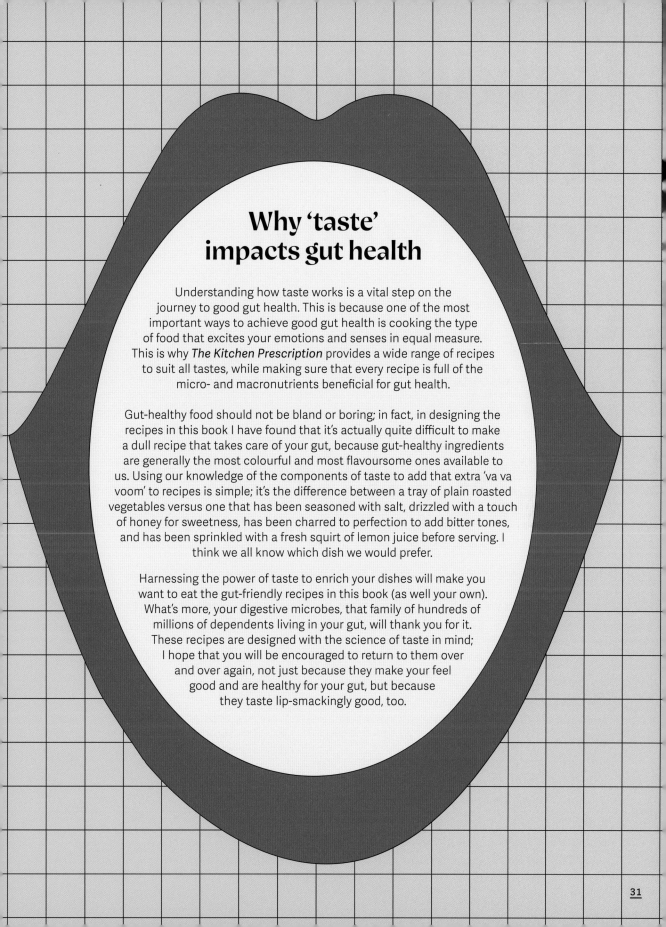

Why 'taste' impacts gut health

Understanding how taste works is a vital step on the journey to good gut health. This is because one of the most important ways to achieve good gut health is cooking the type of food that excites your emotions and senses in equal measure. This is why *The Kitchen Prescription* provides a wide range of recipes to suit all tastes, while making sure that every recipe is full of the micro- and macronutrients beneficial for gut health.

Gut-healthy food should not be bland or boring; in fact, in designing the recipes in this book I have found that it's actually quite difficult to make a dull recipe that takes care of your gut, because gut-healthy ingredients are generally the most colourful and most flavoursome ones available to us. Using our knowledge of the components of taste to add that extra 'va va voom' to recipes is simple; it's the difference between a tray of plain roasted vegetables versus one that has been seasoned with salt, drizzled with a touch of honey for sweetness, has been charred to perfection to add bitter tones, and has been sprinkled with a fresh squirt of lemon juice before serving. I think we all know which dish we would prefer.

Harnessing the power of taste to enrich your dishes will make you want to eat the gut-friendly recipes in this book (as well your own). What's more, your digestive microbes, that family of hundreds of millions of dependents living in your gut, will thank you for it. These recipes are designed with the science of taste in mind; I hope that you will be encouraged to return to them over and over again, not just because they make your feel good and are healthy for your gut, but because they taste lip-smackingly good, too.

Revolutionise your gut health with the three pillar prescription*

So far, you have been introduced
to the microbiome, the important
macronutrients and micronutrients
which we need to maintain our health,
to the processes behind the digestion
of food, and the mechanisms and
science behind how we taste. Now
I want to focus on the three specific
prescriptions through which you can
revolutionise your gut health.

Prescription 1:

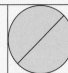

Cook, cook, cook

Cooking is a uniquely human trait: we are the only beings to occupy this earth who can cook. In fact, every known human society today prepares their food by cooking it, which makes it (from an anthropological point of view) an activity which separates human beings from other creatures. There is even a term to describe humans as beings designed to cook what is eaten, derived from the Latin *coquere* (to cook); we are the only 'coctivores' on the planet.

According to a theory suggested by primatologist Richard Wrangham at Harvard University, the act of cooking has played a fundamental transformative role in unlocking the nutrients necessary for us to evolve into the humans we are today. It started around 2 million or so years ago when for the first time in history, eating cooked, energy-dense food (rather than raw, difficult-to-digest food) resulted in the size and complexity of our evolutionary forefathers' brains increasing and the size of their teeth and gut decreasing. So, because of cooking, we have become the clever, sophisticated beings we are today: a humbling thought.

I dwell on these anthropological theories in a book about cooking for gut health for a reason. They prove that cooking is a fundamentally human trait, and therefore we should all be cooking, no excuses. There is also very real evidence that tells us that home cooking is good for health. I know many of you will know this already, intuitively, but there is also evidence to share with the sceptics.

One particularly good study found that those people who ate home-cooked meals more than five times per week were 28 per cent less likely to be overweight when compared with people cooking their meals for less than three days a week. Further evidence across a host of studies has demonstrated that cooking improves mood, self-esteem, confidence and so much more. Although unclear to what extent, there is no denying that at least a part of these described benefits are a consequence of the positive impact that home-cooked food has on the gut microbiome.

By cooking our own food, we avoid intake of shop-bought ultra-processed, highly modified food, with all the added sugar, fat, salt as well as emulsifiers, additives and preservatives that it contains. Food processing alters the structure of food, changing its properties and how it is used by the body. Ultra-processed foods are sadly becoming dominant in our global food system, which is a problem because they are fairly conclusively linked to certain negative metabolic changes.

There is compelling evidence that ultra-processed food (whether from animal or plant sources) is associated with a poorer gut microbiome composition. The PREDICT study has identified that diets with more highly processed plant-based foods and less healthy animal-based foods (e.g. processed meat) were more likely to be associated with higher levels of 15 'bad' gut microbes linked to poorer health markers. In contrast, people who eat a diet rich in less processed plant-based food and healthy animal-based food, e.g., oily fish, eggs and yoghurt, were more likely to have higher levels of 15 'good' gut microbes, linked to markers of good health. The science is telling us that cooking your own food from scratch at home is far superior for your gut health than relying on ultra-processed shop-bought options.

I find it very hard to accept that unless affected by specific impairments to function, people 'just cannot cook'. If we are to foster good gut health it is essential to break away from the 'can't cook, won't cook' attitude. In an ideal world, I would argue that we should all be taught cookery from a young age at school, in order to not only equip us with this most basic survival skill, but also to get us into the mindset of seeing cooking as accessible and simple from the very beginning of a child's journey into adulthood.

For this reason, I would encourage you to cook these recipes with your children where possible, shop for the ingredients with them, and get their input on which recipes they want to try; they will not only understand the basic principles of gut-healthy eating from a young age, but will also have fun with you while they do it. By involving them in your journey towards a healthier gut, you will not only get them interested in eating home-cooked, non-processed yummy food, but you'll also give them a sense of ownership over the finished product.

A helpful task is to work collaboratively with your children in the supermarket to ensure the shopping basket has fruit and vegetables, whole grains, pulses and legumes, seeds and nuts in it every week. This may start as a conscious exercise, but slowly you will notice it becomes subconscious; you just become a gut-healthy shopper. I was particularly delighted in the supermarket the other day when my seven-year-old pointed out that we had forgotten to buy tinned lentils; there are moments of maternal pride, and there are moments of maternal pride.

In this book I have intentionally concentrated on extremely simple methods and techniques. This is how I approach cooking in my own home; simple and nutritious is the mantra that I repeat in my head when I am choosing what to cook for dinner. Even though I won *MasterChef*, my own kitchen is tiny; 2 x 2 metres (not including the cabinets!) with only one small work surface, a gas cooker and a single oven. I don't have space for a sous vide machine or anything more complicated than a food processor, toaster and kettle. I imagine a fair few of you are cooking under similar conditions, and so it was in my best interests that every recipe in this book could be prepared easily in any kitchen, from the most extravagant and well equipped to, well, mine.

One critique of home cooking is that it can end up being more expensive to buy the fresh ingredients required to cook a meal, when compared with the cost of buying ready-made processed frozen meals or opting for takeaway options.

As a young family living in London I am wary of budget and have developed my own money-saving gut-health hacks. For example, I buy the leftover vegetables in the discount corner of the supermarket; I use tinned pulses and frozen vegetables galore in my recipes; and I use far less meat than you might expect. All these things help save the pennies. I am also a meticulous meal planner, and I encourage this as a way of maximising the opportunities to cook gut-healthy meals in the week. I use the following tool to plan my weekly shop and minimise wastage. I have shared my template here as it may be of some use to you too.

Weekly Food Plan

Monday	*Gut-healing Masala Cottage Pie*	**Existing storecupboard ingredients to use up**
Tuesday	*Good Gut Tacos*	• Tinned mango • Pearl barley • Tinned chickpeas
Wednesday	*Za'atar Lasagne Verde*	**Ingredients to buy**
Thursday		• Fresh fruit and vegetables • Tinned goods • Frozen food • Other • Treat of the week
Friday		
Saturday		
Sunday		

As the child of a full-time working mother who took pride in feeding her three children freshly cooked meals daily, I can confirm that it is not always easy to build cooking into our 21st-century whirlwind lives: it takes a bit of time and experimentation to establish a rhythm and style that works well for you. It took me a few years to work out how to do it properly and I am still not sure how my mother managed it all. But I also know that the home-cooked meals I was lucky enough to eat with my family at the dinner table – with all the bickering and knocking elbows that involved – were vital for my cognitive development, physical health and mental wellbeing. Those meals have literally and figuratively made me the person I am today. I hope that you can be convinced that being prescribed 'cooking' will enrich not just your gut bugs, but your life as a whole.

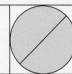

Prescription 2:

Feed your gut bugs

You already understand what your gut microbiome is and what it does, so it is time to understand what we can do to help the inhabitants of our gut. You should, by now, have figured out that the food we eat has a direct influence on the composition of our gut microbiota. What you may not know is that over the years we have been reducing the variety of food that we feed our helpful little gut friends.

For example, by studying petrified poos and stomachs we know that 15,000 years ago people would eat more than 150 ingredients per week, whereas most of us now eat fewer than 20. Of the over 250,000 known edible species of plant on earth we use fewer than 200, and if you think that's bad wait until you find out that *three-quarters of the food we consume globally comes from just five animal and 12 plant species.*

I've already mentioned how eating more plant-based foods as part of a diverse diet will make a positive difference to your microbiota. But another more focused way of cultivating the microbiota in your gut is to treat it to a diet rich in prebiotic and probiotic foods.

Prebiotics

Prebiotics are a bit like the Miracle-Gro we apply to our lawn, in that they fertilise the bowel and encourage the growth and proliferation of the microbiota in your gut. Prebiotics are rich in fibre, which we would be unable to digest if it were not for our microbiota. Our gut microbes break fibre down to release a chemical called butyrate, which plays a key role in keeping the gut wall healthy and helps to maintain the function of the gut barrier (a complicated structure which allows nutrients and immune cells into the body, but keeps pathogens and harmful things out), as well as decreasing inflammation.

Some popular and readily available prebiotics include the following: whole grains, apples, bananas, leeks, asparagus, dandelion greens, cauliflower, broccoli, Jerusalem artichokes, chicory, honey, garlic, seeds, nuts, lentils, dried mango, prunes, grapefruit, cocoa and green tea extracts. You may have noticed that these foods are plant-based; I have intentionally used many of them in the recipes in this book. Just try to build up the amount of prebiotic ingredients in your diet slowly, as sudden increases in prebiotic fibre can shock the inhabitants of your gut and result in unpleasant bloating. Slow and steady wins the gut health race!

Current guidelines suggest that we consume 30g of fibre a day (see table below), but in reality, most people fall far short of this most of the time. Although fibre is an intrinsic part of any good diet (because plant-based foods like fruits and vegetables, whole grains, nuts and seeds, legumes and pulses are naturally dense in fibre), in nutrition terms it is not technically an 'essential nutrient'; strictly speaking, a fibre deficiency does not exist.

Ingredient	Total fibre per 100g
Wholewheat or bran cereals	13–24.5g
Wholemeal bread (2 slices)	7g
Wholemeal spaghetti (cooked)	4.2g
Figs	6.9g
Strawberries	3.8g
Parsnip (boiled)	4.7g
Broccoli (boiled)	2.8g
Almonds	7.4g
Peanuts	7.6g
Sesame seeds	7.9g
Sunflower seeds	6.0g
Peas (boiled)	5.6g
Baked beans	4.9g
Green beans (boiled)	4.1g
Chia seeds	35g
Haricot beans	11g

Fibre can be divided into two groups: soluble and insoluble. Soluble fibres dissolve in water, for example plant pectins. In contrast, insoluble fibres such as plant cellulose don't dissolve in water. Most plants contain both soluble and insoluble fibre components in different amounts, but oats, beans and fruits are higher sources of soluble fibre while wheat, nuts, seeds, bran, fruit skins and legumes are richer in insoluble fibre. Because, as mentioned earlier, the only place both types of fibre can be broken down in the body is the colon, it's important that we keep the bacteria that carry out this role in tip-top condition.

Fibre consumption has been fairly conclusively linked to a reduction in heart disease, type 2 diabetes, stroke and colorectal cancer. Some studies go as far as saying that for every 8g increase in dietary fibre per day, the risk of total deaths and incidence of these ailments can decrease by up to 19 per cent. So whether you are eating more plant-based foods, making a conscious effort to maximise fibre intake or consuming more prebiotics, it all amounts to the same thing: you will be optimising gut microbial diversity through tasty food, with the added benefit of preventing a multitude of non-communicable diseases.

Probiotics

While prebiotics are food for the bacteria that live inside us, probiotic foods actually contain live bacteria. These bacteria have been produced by the process of lacto-fermentation; the theory is that when we eat probiotic foods, these bacteria will, given the right conditions, find their way into the bowel, make a nice cosy home and have lots of cute little bacteria babies. I say theory, because there is very little research confirming whether the various available probiotics contain enough bacteria to be effective. In the UK, probiotics are actually classified as food rather than medicine and are labelled as having 'live bacteria or cultures' as opposed to 'probiotic'. This is simply because there is no guarantee that the required number of beneficial bacteria will be consumed and reach the large bowel alive.

Probiotics are not, therefore, some sort of miraculous gut-curing superfood. However, at worst they're pretty harmless, and there's a good chance that they may do you some good (plus, they taste great, so it's kind of a win-win situation for you and your gut). I personally love their slightly acidic taste and characteristic sweet smell, but I get that these are acquired tastes. With time and practice you might learn to love probiotics too.

What we don't know is whether natural probiotics in food are better for gut health than probiotic supplements. Personally, I would much rather you experimented with probiotic foods in your kitchen than spent money on probiotic supplements in the form of tablets or drinks which carry with them variable evidence for effectiveness

A note on probiotic foods:

As discussed, these foods have all been produced by the process of fermentation, which is an art form that I am passionate about. In many ways our fridges have changed the way we eat. We always look at the sell by date of food and have fallen into the mindset that bacteria on food is synonymous with danger, but this is not always the case. There is actually a world of bacteria out there that are usually completely innocuous and often quite beneficial.

I find a real sense of pleasure in the process of fermentation; it gives me a connection to creation and increases my familiarity with the process of decay, something we tend to avoid these days. I would urge you all to have a go at fermenting in your spare time, whether that is fermentation of spare vegetables that would otherwise go to waste, or playing around with a sourdough starter.

See some examples of fermented foods on the next page.

8 popular lacto-fermented foods that you can try

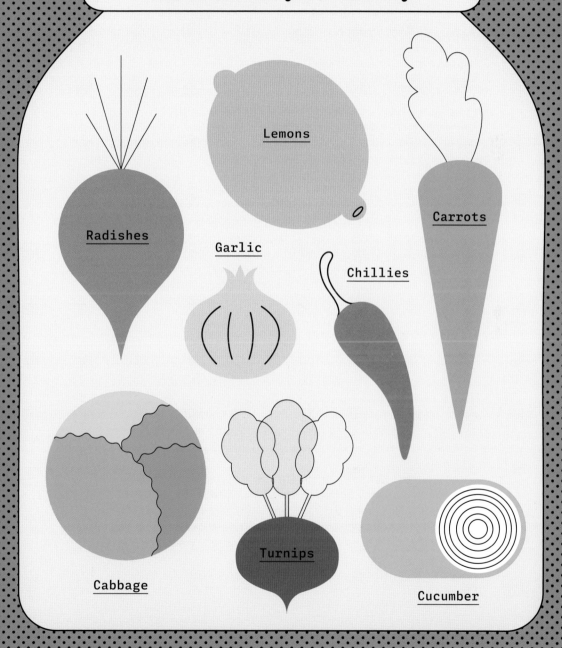

Lemons

Radishes

Garlic

Chillies

Carrots

Cabbage

Turnips

Cucumber

Here are some examples of probiotic foods you can experiment with:

☐ **Sauerkraut:** This dish of shredded raw cabbage fermented in brine by various lactic acid bacteria is popular across Eastern and Central Europe. The cabbage is rubbed vigorously with salt before being packed into a jar with its briny juices. You can add various seasonings like caraway, juniper berries, pink peppercorns or fennel (among others). I love using some red and white cabbage together as it gives a pretty coloured sauerkraut that looks very appealing. If you want to give sauerkraut a try, see **page 80** for my **Egg and Sauerkraut Mayo on Rye**.

☐ **Kimchi:** There are literally hundreds of varieties of this Korean fermented dish. It is made from the leaves of Chinese leaf which are seasoned with various spices, including garlic, ginger or dried shrimp before being packed away to ferment. The Koreans love it so much that they have a museum dedicated to kimchi in Seoul; the average person eats a massive 26kg of it annually, so I guess the museum is pretty popular too. Kimchi is probably my favourite fermented dish of all time, and definitely worth trying in my recipe for **Kimchi and Garlic Fried Rice** on **page 160**.

☐ **Yoghurt:** Not all yoghurts contain live cultures, so be wary when you are buying your weekly tub. I have used live yoghurt throughout the recipes featured in this book, mostly because I just love the taste. If you do buy a 'live' yoghurt and have some time to spare, then you can actually use that live yoghurt as a starter culture to make more yoghurt. Simply heat 1 litre (2 pints) of full-fat milk to 82°C (180°F), allow it to cool to 46°C (115°F) and then add a tablespoon of starter culture at room temperature. The yoghurt needs to be kept at 43–46°C (109–115°F) for 3–8 hours until it sets (a thermostat-controlled oven or airing cupboard are good places for this). Once set, store it in the fridge and enjoy within a couple of days.

☐ **Kefir:** Kefir is a cultured, fermented milk drink that tastes a little bit fizzy and a little bit sour. It works well in desserts, like my recipe for **Blackberry Kefir Panna Cotta** on **page 240**. Kefir also pairs equally well with a variety of fruit in summery smoothies; see my **Refreshing Kefir, Raspberry and Rose Cooler** on **page 54**.

☐ **Kombucha:** This is a fermented drink made from a sweetened tea and a specific culture called a SCOBY (Symbiotic Culture of Bacteria and Yeasts). Many fruity, spiced and floral versions are available to try in supermarkets these days. Try my recipe for **Kombucha, Raspberry and Elderflower Jelly** on **page 244**.

☐ **Labneh:** This is a really thick, luscious, slightly tangy tasting Middle Eastern strained yoghurt cheese. You can make a version of it by hanging Greek yoghurt in a cheesecloth overnight in the fridge, with a bowl underneath to catch all the water that drips out. Alternatively, you can buy it from Middle Eastern food shops in tubs that look like Philadelphia cream cheese, or even jarred and flavoured with herbs like mint and parsley and steeped in olive oil. See my recipe for **Sunshine Tomatoes and Labneh on Toast** on **page 62** or for those special moments try my **Labneh, Passion Fruit and Ginger Cheesecake** on **page 234**.

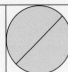

Prescription 3:

Do not diet

Let's cut to the chase: if you are trying to lose weight, restrictive diets do not work.

That's not to say that many structured diet plans do initially result in rapid weight loss. However, what they don't tell you is that this is usually followed by a weight plateau and then rapid weight gain. A meta-analysis (where researchers combine the results of lots of similar studies to get a wider view of what is going on) of 29 long-term weight-loss studies was performed. Meta-analysis is considered the very best type of scientific evidence, and this meta-analysis was pretty telling; more than half of the lost weight on these diet programmes was regained within two years, and by five years more than 80 per cent of lost weight was regained (see below).

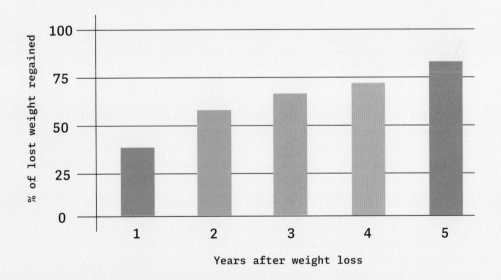

Years after weight loss

Another large meta-analysis looked at 121 trials that enrolled around 22,000 overweight or obese adults who were following one of 14 popular diets, including Atkins, Weight Watchers, Jenny Craig, DASH (Dietary Approaches to Stop Hypertension) and others, for an average of six months. Although the diets showed a reduction in blood pressure and weight at six months, by twelve months the weight reduction and improvements in cardiovascular risk factors had vanished.

I have first-hand experience of many patients who describe the peaks and troughs on their weight-loss journey. One patient of mine, a 49-year-old NHS secretary, was suffering with high blood pressure, borderline diabetes and high cholesterol for years. A year earlier, she had started a popular weight-loss programme and lost an astonishing 15kg of weight. Not only this, but her blood pressure and cholesterol had improved, and she was no longer a borderline diabetic. This was, according to her, the happiest and healthiest she had felt since her teenage years.

For one reason or another, as is so common with such diets, this patient was unable to keep up with the programme. Within eight months of stopping, she had gained back all the weight she had lost. She came to my clinic after developing a skin infection from a mosquito bite on her leg, devastated that her health had declined so much. She genuinely believed that there was no programme on the planet that would allow her to lose weight, and importantly to keep it off for good. With her wedding coming up in the summer, she was desperate to shed the pounds and sort out her health once and for all.

I recall having an open discussion with this patient about the factors that she felt led to her gaining weight after losing it. How many of these can you relate to?

+ She described the office environment where she worked, where everyone took turns to bring in extremely delicious (but extremely processed) snacks, snacks full of salt, sugar and fat and designed to arouse our primal urge for these tastes.

+ She felt that 'calorie counting' did more harm than good. For her, the 1,800–2,000kcal a day target was becoming a source of immense stress, bound with feelings of failure when she went past the target, cementing the idea that she was not in control of her eating.

+ She found that working to a set number of calories per day was so irritating and restrictive that she was prone to rebelling against the rules of the diet. She described one evening where, angry at herself for eating more than her calorie allowance that day, she went through a whole tub of ice cream in front of the TV.

I'd hazard a guess that anyone who has tried any kind of restrictive diet can empathise with all three of these complaints. The irony of the matter is that even though the 'less calories equals less weight' idea has been drilled into us from the moment we were old enough to pick up a parents' magazine or watch a beauty ad on TV, the concept of whether counting calories is helpful is the subject of much debate in nutrition circles. Food is so much more than calories, and reducing it down to a mere number risks oversimplifying the nourishment and non-calorie benefit that food can provide. More than that, what a calorie is to my body may not be the same as what a calorie is for your body, so I suggest taking any calorie-counting advice with a healthy pinch of salt.

The most recent research is showing us that more than calories, it is the composition of the microbiome that might be responsible for the huge variances in how different people process sugars and other nutrients in foods, which means that the composition of the gut microbiome may also play a role in weight gain and the development of obesity. So, rather than focusing on the number of calories consumed, try focusing on introducing enough variety of food into your daily diet, and on fostering good microbial diversity within your gut.

For my patient, it was a huge conceptual shift to move away from a restrictive weight-loss journey, to one that placed the diversity of her microbiota as the main priority. To her indoctrinated mind, if it didn't feel like suffering, then it didn't feel like dieting. But – and I cannot stress this enough – it is the restrictive parts of any weight-loss programme, the ones that make us feel like we are suffering, that make people fail on these diet plans in the first place. Instead, the evidence suggests that doctors should be trying to focus their patients on eating a diverse array of foods over the course of a week, foods which include as many different plant-based food groups as possible. Only then we will be doing them, and their gut, a real favour.

Throughout *The Kitchen Prescription*, you will see that the inclusion of food groups is the focus, rather than exclusion of particular foods from the diet. Food diversity really does matter when pursuing good gut health; studies have shown that eating 30 plant species a week is linked to the production of various short-chain fatty acids, which help to protect both our gut health and strengthen our immune systems, and it can also foster a varied internal microbial community. Do you think you reach this target of 30 plant species?

So forget about calories and instead focus on eating the rainbow. Add colour to each and every plate you eat. It's a lot easier to think about whether you have eaten green, red, purple and orange foods this week than to think about how many calories were in those chips or whether you have enough calories left for a slice of pizza or a second helping of dinner. Not only are colourful plant foods rich in fibre, they are also chock-full of polyphenols, those antioxidant compounds that the 'good' gut microbes love. So every way you look at it, brightly coloured fruit and veg is good for you.

As a physician, I feel the best approach is to support and encourage patients to make small, piecemeal, but sustainable improvements. Nobody in their right mind expects you to incorporate 30 plant species a week in your diet immediately; that is unrealistic, but more importantly it's unsustainable. Take the time to assess roughly how many different plants you already consume each week (fruit and vegetables, whole grains, nuts and seeds, beans and pulses, herbs and spices, that sort of thing) and then slowly but steadily build up the diversity in your diet, allowing the gut time to adjust to each new array of goodness. (Doing it too rapidly can result in excessive bloating and discomfort.) Remember, it's a marathon, not a sprint.

Some people I have met find it helpful to keep a **Plant diversity checklist** where they tally the number of different plant-based foods they are eating over the course of the week. It is quite satisfying to see the tally count gradually extending week on week and even more satisfying to hear about all the beneficial effects that eating a diverse diet has on an individual's health and wellbeing. Try this tallying exercise if this is something that you feel would work for you.

I have developed a **Plant diversity score** for each recipe in the book. This can be seen in the top lefthand corner of each recipe. This score awards each portion of fruit and vegetable, wholegrain, legume, pulse, nut and seed one plant diversity point. Herbs, spices and condiments score a quarter of a plant diversity point, so if four or more spices are used in a recipe, they add up to a single plant diversity point. As a rough guide the higher your weekly plant diversity score, the better.

Add the recipes featured in this book gradually into your kitchen repertoire and remember that these gut-focused recipes are part of a broader picture, where good sleep and physical activity also play a vital part. There will be times when you slip up but don't beat yourself up when it happens. Just take it one step at a time and with every step forward that you take, be content in the knowledge that you are one step closer to a healthy gut.

I like to think that through the food I choose, I am, in fact, communicating directly with my gut bugs, nourishing them, creating a comfortable environment for them, and allowing them to thrive; in turn, they are helping me to flourish. Revolutionising gut health is perhaps as much about feeding our gut bugs as it is about feeding ourselves, but with a bit of practice we can do both of these things successfully with minimal effort.

A diverse gut microbiome has in some ways become synonymous with good health these days, but there is a way to go before we can say with certainty what the optimal way of achieving gut health is. For now, what we can say is that steadily incorporating more plant-based (fruit and vegetables, whole grains, legumes and pulses, seeds and nuts), fibre-rich foods, prebiotics, probiotics (if you fancy them), and some tasty bug-laden fermented foods into your diet will give you the highest chance of success in improving your gut health.

I wish you and your gut bugs the best of luck on your journey. Now, on to the recipes!

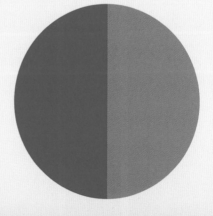

Plant diversity checklist

	Week One	Week Two
1	Apple	Sprouts
2	Orange	Rocket
3	Barley	Melon
4	Rice	Plums
5	Corn	Chilli
6	Kiwi	Pineapple
7		Aubergine
8		Carrots
9		
10		
11		
12		
13		
14		
15		
16		
17		
18		
19		
20		
21		
22		
23		
24		
25		
26		
27		
28		
29		
30		
31		

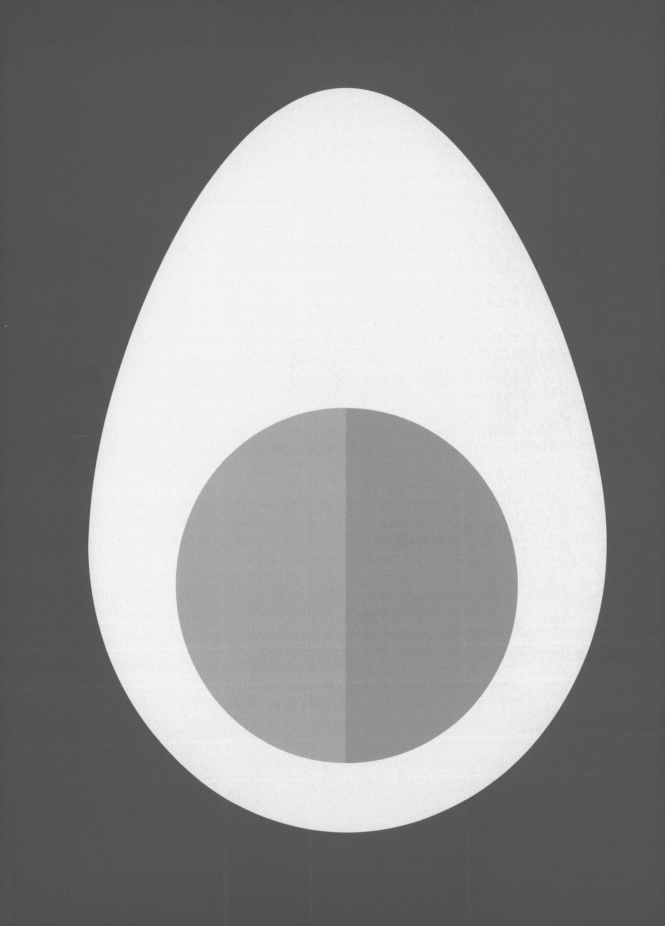

BREAKFAST

Gut morning...

My partner and I are fairly similar in our meal habits. However, we have two opposing breakfast rituals. Breakfast excites me so much that sometimes I'll give up a lie-in just to try something new. My husband, on the other hand, literally couldn't care less. And yet, here we both are, both very much alive and healthy. So, what's the truth behind breakfast? Is it really 'the most important meal of the day'? Or is that just another deceitful dietary dogma?

The trouble is that over the years the messaging swings from one extreme to the other, it is a pendulum that never stops. One minute we are ingrained to believe that eating breakfast is vital for our metabolic health and is the single most important meal of the day. The next moment intermittent fasting and skipping breakfast is in vogue.

If you're confused, take solace in the fact that you're not alone. Many nutrition experts are bewildered by the conflicting messages surrounding breakfast. The reason that nobody can make their minds up about breakfast is, quite simply, that nobody has ALL the answers (and you should treat anyone who says they do with a healthy dose of scepticism).

Nutrition is never black and white, and because of the sheer number of variables that scientists have to account for, studying the impact of breakfast on a person's weight, health and overall wellbeing is, well, complicated. These variables are ably demonstrated by me and my husband.

While on any given day we might both have breakfast, what we choose to eat will differ, the time in the morning we eat it will differ, how large our breakfast is compared to our lunch and dinner will differ. Even family structure, socio-economic background and ethnicity have been shown to have an impact on the health benefits of breakfast. And because breakfast isn't some identical lump of food ingested at exactly 6.30 a.m. by everyone on earth, its effect on health can differ from person to person.

Most recently, a multitude of studies have discredited the perceived disadvantages of skipping breakfast; overall, combining all the data, it seems that there is no evidence to support the claim that skipping breakfast makes you gain weight. Additionally, a concept which is enjoying a growing consensus among scientists and nutritionists is that a regular meal pattern, i.e., where you eat meals at roughly the same time each day, is a good thing. Because we are all governed by a natural circadian rhythm' a body clock which influences when we wake and sleep, the time we have our meals has been shown to influence this pattern.

The trillions of gut microbes living within us may also have their own circadian rhythm, varying in composition and function when fasting versus when fed. Early evidence even suggests that short periods of fasting (like skipping breakfast) might even be beneficial for the gut microbiome; this is an evolving area of research which we will surely learn more about in years to come.

Some people are programmed to prefer eating food early in the morning while others prefer a later start. There is no one way that works for everyone; we need to respect the fact that many lack the desire or appetite for breakfast. For me, what you choose to eat for breakfast matters more than whether or not you eat it. There is such thing as a 'good' breakfast and a 'bad' breakfast.

Breakfast options have come a long way since an entire country was trained to eat cereal, toasted sliced white bread and fruit juice every morning. There is now a vast world of more exciting plant-powered, microbe-rich, gut-fuelling, cross-cultural breakfast options to choose from – or indeed to cook.

The recipes in this chapter are bursting with flavour and are light, bright and refreshing and designed to incorporate both prebiotics and probiotics (pages 36–40). I feel breakfast is a strategic opportunity to optimise gut health and many breakfast foods are naturally designed to restore gut health; think dependable, affordable oats, satisfying tangy kefir, creamy live yoghurt or the pure macro- and micronutrient-filled goodness of fruits, nuts and seeds. This opportunity shouldn't be wasted. I've listed the recipes that follow as breakfast recipes but really, you can pamper your gut with these dishes at any time of the day.

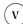

Fig, Date + Seed Yoghurt

SERVES 4

Plant Diversity
Score: 3

This breakfast is as gut loving as it gets. Figs, dates and sunflower seeds are a rich source of fibre and live Greek yoghurt is probiotic. If you are vegan, replace the Greek yoghurt with a thick-set plant-based yoghurt of your choice. I use both fresh and dried varieties of fig in this recipe, but if fresh figs are not in season, you can use any other fresh seasonal fruit you have to hand.

—

7 dried figs, roughly chopped

150g (5oz) chopped pitted dates

2 tbsp sunflower seeds

200ml (7fl oz/generous ¾ cup) kettle-hot water

300g (10oz) full-fat live Greek yoghurt (or plant-based yoghurt)

6 fresh figs, thinly sliced

1. Place the dried figs, dates, half the sunflower seeds and the hot water in a blender and blitz to a smooth purée. Allow the mixture to cool to room temperature, then combine this cooled fig and date mixture with the Greek yoghurt and toss in the remaining sunflower seeds. (I do this as I quite like the textural variation you get when using whole seeds.)

2. Place the yoghurt in a wide, shallow bowl. Top with the sliced figs, creating a bit of a pattern with slightly overlapping fig slices. This is not essential, but does look rather appealing.

3. This will keep well in the fridge for a few days.

— the kitchen prescription

Figs (Ficus carica)

+ Figs are rich in polyphenols, compounds with protective antioxidant properties that help us to repair damaged tissues and act as fuel for our gut microbes.

+ Figs are rich in a number of minerals (particularly calcium, potassium, copper, iron and magnesium) as well as vitamin B6.

+ The very high fibre content of figs means that they act as a natural laxative: they have long been used as a home remedy for constipation.

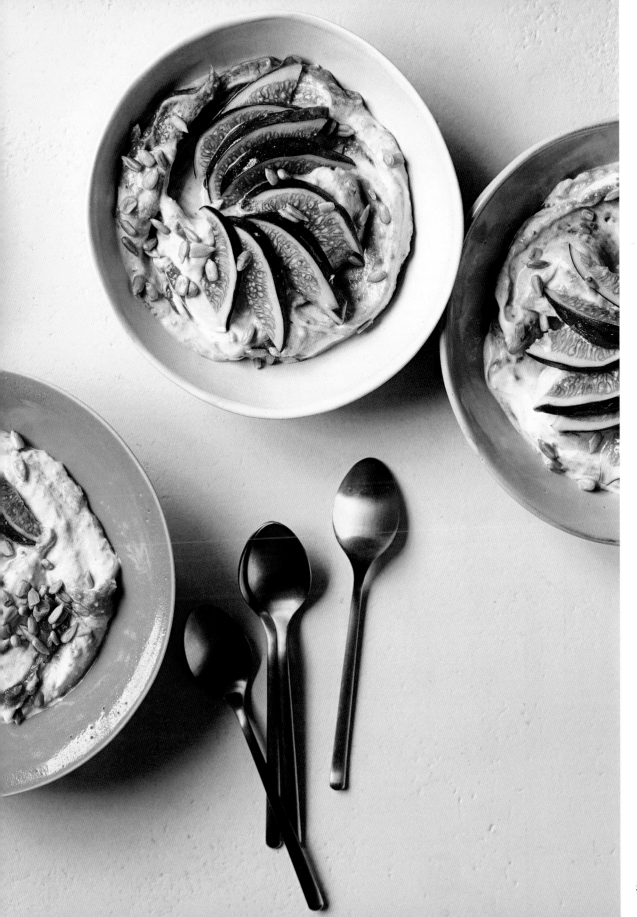

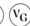

Mango + Chia Seed Pudding

SERVES 4

Plant Diversity
Score: 3.5

In this recipe the chia seeds swell and magically thicken the mango and coconut milk mixture. The seeds themselves have very little flavour of their own; they are, however, excellent sponges for added fruity flavours, which is how I would recommend you use them at breakfast. Handily, this dish keeps incredibly well in the fridge for a few days, so you can keep some for the next day's breakfast. If you can't get hold of tinned mango pulp, just blitz up some tinned or fresh mango in a blender to create a home-made mango pulp instead.

—

1 x 400ml (14fl oz) tin full-fat organic coconut milk

1 tbsp maple syrup

200ml (7fl oz/generous ¾ cup) tinned mango pulp/purée

¼ tsp ground cardamom (or the seeds of 3 crushed pods)

½ tsp fennel seeds, crushed in a pestle and mortar

Zest and juice of 1 lime

75g (2¾oz/½ cup) chia seeds

1. Combine all the ingredients, except the chia seeds, in a bowl and whisk well to combine. You want to make sure that any coconut solids are well emulsified into the mixture and no lumps remain.

2. Add the chia seeds and stir gently for a minute or two. You will notice the mixture will start to thicken. Place it in the fridge for a few hours before serving. (You can also make this the night before for breakfast the next morning.)

3. Top with a dollop of Greek yoghurt and fruit of your choice.

BONUS GUT-FRIENDLY TOPPINGS

1 dollop of full-fat live Greek yoghurt or plant-based yoghurt of your choice

Handful of fresh or tinned mango chunks or other fruit, e.g. passion fruit

the kitchen prescription

Chia seeds (seeds of the plant Salvia hispanica L.)

+ There is emerging evidence that chia seeds may be beneficial to heart health and help to lower blood pressure. They are rich in polyunsaturated omega-3 fatty acids.

+ Chia seeds are thought to exert a beneficial effect on insulin resistance and blood sugar responses.

+ They are a rich source of fibre, and this may be beneficial for our gut

microbiome. A 25g (1oz) portion of chia seeds contains about 9g (⅓oz) of fibre, just under a third of our recommended daily fibre intake.

+ There is no doubt that chia seeds have beneficial effects on health. However, they can be added by marketing departments to less nutritious foods, in order to improve a product's appeal to 'health conscious' consumers. Be wary!

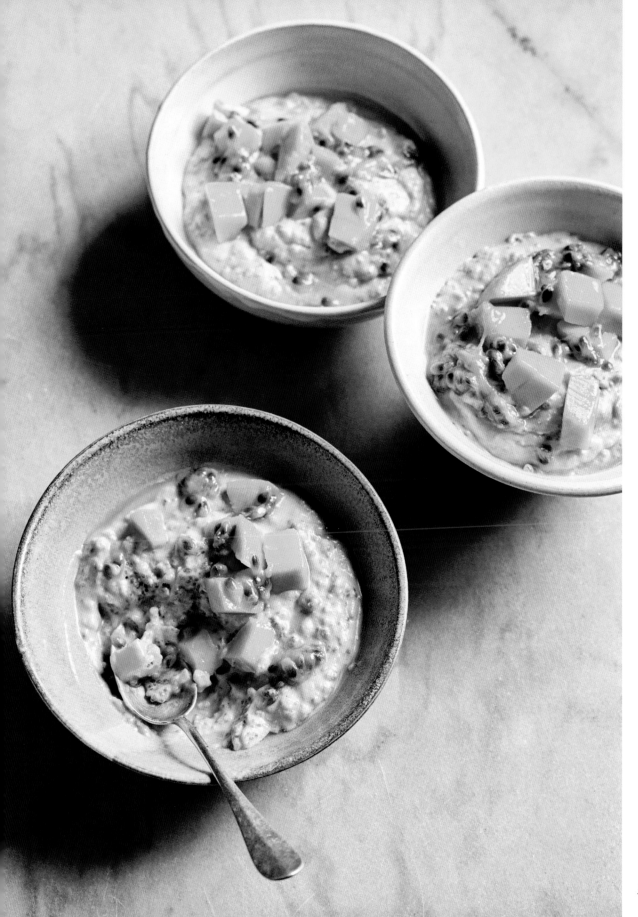

Refreshing Kefir, Raspberry + Rose Cooler

SERVES 2

Plant Diversity
Score: 1.25

If you're after a refreshing sip on a warm summer day, the lactic tang of kefir in this recipe works perfectly against the tart sweetness of seedy raspberries and perfume of rosewater. I use raspberries because they are a rich source of vitamin C, which helps support the immune system; they are also thought to help collagen production in the skin. Just a cup of raspberries has about 8g (⅓oz) of fibre – more than many other fruits.

—

200g (7oz) raspberries
(fresh or frozen)

3–4 ice cubes

1–2 tsp rosewater
(not rose extract)

1 tbsp maple syrup or honey

½ tsp fennel seeds

500ml (16fl oz/2 cups) kefir

1. Place the raspberries, ice, rosewater, maple syrup, fennel seeds and a quarter of the kefir in a blender and blitz until very smooth. The amount of rosewater you use will depend on the quality the rosewater that you have and also how floral you like your drink.

2. Pour the remaining kefir into the blended raspberry mixture and stir to combine. Serve immediately.

the kitchen prescription

Kefir

+ A cultured fermented probiotic milk drink that was first made in the mountainous regions between Asia and Europe. Carbon dioxide, a by-product of the fermentation process, gives the kefir a slight fizzy note.

+ Depending on the variety used, it can contain over 30 strains of beneficial bacteria and yeasts. The starter culture comes in the shape of a grain called a SCOBY (Symbiotic Colony of Bacteria and Yeast).

+ Kefir is an excellent source of complete amino acids and calcium, which is important for bone health.

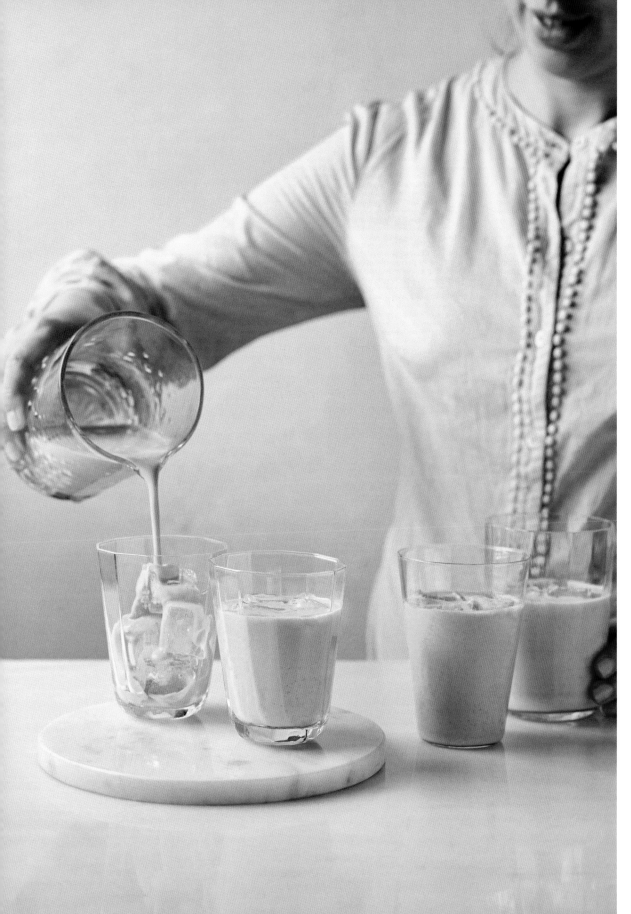

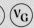

Piña Colada Baked Oats

SERVES 6

Plant Diversity
Score: 3
Bonus Score: 1

Now, pineapple and coconut might sound a bit odd for breakfast, maybe more suited to a tall glass on a beach, but on a blank oaty canvas the flavour combination is actually very pleasing. Even better, by baking the oats you remove the need to stand at the stove stirring a pot of oats till your arm feels as if it will drop off. You might find yourself fighting your children or spouse for the golden crusty parts that form on the surface as the dish bakes, so be prepared to slap away some thieving hands.

—

200g (7oz/2 cups) rolled oats (or gluten-free rolled oats)

1 x 400ml (14fl oz) tin full-fat organic coconut milk

400ml (14fl oz) semi-skimmed milk (or plant-based milk)

75g (2¾oz) grated fresh coconut or desiccated coconut

250g (9oz) fresh pineapple, cut into small chunks (or 1 x 425g/15oz tin pineapple, drained weight 250g/9oz)

1 heaped tbsp demerara sugar

BONUS GUT-FRIENDLY TOPPINGS

For extra flavour and texture add a handful of nuts or seeds, e.g. almonds or sunflower seeds

1. Preheat the oven to 180°C fan/ 200°C/gas mark 6.

2. Combine all the ingredients in a ceramic or porcelain pie dish. Bake in the oven for 30–40 minutes, sprinkling the sugar over the top of the dish for the last 10–15 minutes or so of baking. This will allow a nice golden crust to form. Serve immediately with a handful of nuts or seeds for extra flavour and texture if you like.

Choco-nut Porridge

SERVES 1

Plant Diversity
Score: 2.25
Bonus Score: 1

60g (2½oz/¾ cup) porridge oats

1 tbsp good-quality cocoa powder

1 heaped tsp almond butter (or peanut butter)

200ml (7fl oz/generous ¾ cup) whole milk (use plant based milk if you prefer)

Honey or maple syrup, to sweeten

1 tbsp toasted flaked almonds

BONUS GUT-FRIENDLY TOPPINGS

Sliced banana or a few roughly chopped prunes

This one is a real children pleaser and far better for their little guts than a bowl of chocolate-flavoured processed cereal. I make this in the microwave for ease, but you can just as easily make it in a big batch on the stove.

—

1. Combine the oats, cocoa powder and almond butter in a deep microwave-safe bowl (the almond butter won't mix in with remaining ingredients at this stage). Add the milk and stir everything well.

2. Microwave on high for 3 minutes, or until the milk has been absorbed. (Note that oat varieties can differ in the amount of liquid they absorb, so if the mixture looks too thick, loosen with an extra splash of milk.) Sweeten with honey or maple syrup to taste.

3. Stir thoroughly and serve topped with the flaked almonds. Add sliced banana or chopped prunes for an extra gut boost.

BREAKFAST

the kitchen prescription

Oats (Avena sativa)

+ Oat kernels that have their outer tough shell removed are called 'oat groats'. These oat groats are then processed in different ways.

+ Steel-cut oats are just the oat groat chopped into smaller pieces with a large steel blade: they are the least processed. Rolled oats are made when oat groats are steamed and flattened. Instant oats are rolled oats that are processed yet further to soften them and reduce cooking time.

+ Oats are a particularly good source of beta-glucans, which are soluble fibres that slow down the absorption of carbohydrates into the bloodstream and therefore prevent spikes in blood sugar.

+ Oats can help lower cholesterol.

+ Oats are a rich source of magnesium, an important mineral that plays a role in over 300 enzyme reactions in the body and supports muscle and nerve function.

57

Gutlicious Granola

SERVES 8

Plant Diversity
Score: 4.5
Bonus Score: 1

This granola is utterly addictive. Packed full of oats, nuts and seeds it is an excellent source of prebiotic dietary fibre. I use powdered jaggery to sweeten this granola – it has a rich, malty, caramelised taste. You should be able to find powdered jaggery in the world food section of your local supermarket, but you can just as easily use soft light brown sugar instead.

—

200g (7oz/2 cups) jumbo rolled oats

150g (5oz) pecans

75g (2¾oz/½ cup) pumpkin seeds

75g (2¾oz/½ cup) sunflower seeds

50g (2oz) powdered jaggery (or soft light brown sugar)

2 tbsp sunflower oil

4 tbsp maple syrup

½ tsp ground cardamom (or the seeds of 6 crushed pods)

½ tsp grated nutmeg

Pinch of salt

BONUS GUT-FRIENDLY TOPPINGS

100g (3½oz/⅔ cup) dried fruit, e.g. sour cherries, dried apricots and/or raisins

1. Preheat the oven to 180°C fan/200°C/gas mark 6 and line a large baking sheet with baking paper.

2. Combine all the ingredients in a large bowl and mix together. Scatter evenly over the baking sheet, transfer to the oven and bake for about 15 minutes, stirring once or twice to ensure that the cereal colours evenly.

3. Remove from the oven and allow to cool before scattering over the dried fruit. Stored in an airtight container or jar, this will keep well for a few weeks.

the kitchen prescription

Jaggery

+ Jaggery is a richer source of micronutrients than refined sugar and is therefore referred to by some as 'medicinal sugar'.

+ It has a slightly lower sucrose content (high-quality jaggery is 70 per cent sucrose) when compared with refined white sugar (99.7 per cent sucrose).

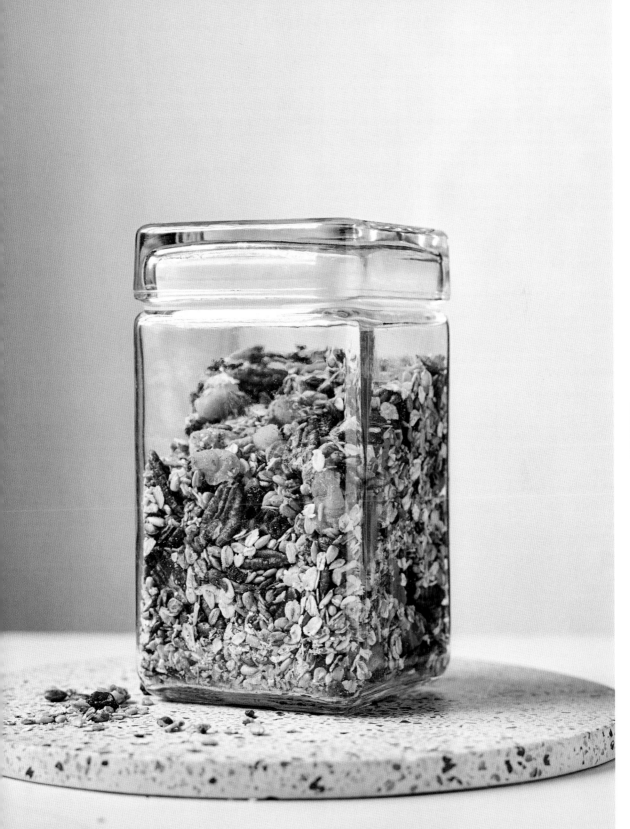

Toast: Three Ways for Three Days

<u>SERVES 1</u>

Plant Diversity
Score: 4; 3.5; 3

Us bread loving Brits consume over 63 billion slices of bread every year. But despite our love for the loaf, research suggests that around two thirds of us wish the item was healthier and had more nutritional benefits. There is a solution. Substitute your regular toast toppings for these gut-friendly ones.

Each topping is designed for 2 slices of toasted seeded sourdough, rye or wholewheat bread.

Topping 1: Peanut Butter + Fresh Chia Berry Jam

1 tbsp crunchy peanut butter

120g (4oz) fresh raspberries

1 tbsp chia seeds

2 tsp honey or maple syrup

Spread the peanut butter over your 2 slices of toast. Crush the berries, chia seeds and maple syrup together in a small bowl. Spoon this coarse-crushed berry and seed mixture over the peanut butter-laden toast. A gut-healthy version of the classic PBJ sandwich.

Topping 2: Cucumber, Pink Radish + Dill

7cm (3in) chunk of cucumber

2 pink radishes

2 tbsp cream cheese

1 tsp finely chopped dill (or any other leftover herbs)

Drizzle of extra-virgin olive oil

Spritz of lemon juice

Salt and pepper, to taste

Slice the cucumber and radishes into very thin rounds. Spread the cream cheese over the 2 slices of toast, then top with the cucumber and radish. Scatter over the dill, drizzle with olive oil and lemon juice, and top with salt and pepper.

Topping 3: Strawberry, Pistachio + Mascarpone

2 tbsp mascarpone (or any cream cheese)

5 strawberries, thinly sliced

Handful of roughly chopped pistachios

Drizzle of maple syrup or honey

Spread the mascarpone cheese over your 2 slices of toast. Top with the strawberries and pistachios. Drizzle with honey or maple syrup to finish.

the kitchen prescription

Bread

My key tips when choosing a gut-friendly loaf are as follows:

+ Choose a loaf made from a wholegrain, unrefined flour, including wholewheat, rye and spelt (it's worth checking the labelling).

+ Try fibre-dense gut-friendly varieties of bread, like German pumpernickel bread, Irish soda bread or Ezekiel bread made from sprouted whole grains.

+ Avoid bread that contains sweeteners and palm oil.

+ Sourdough has undergone a long process of fermentation. This increases the availability of various vitamins, minerals and polyphenolic compounds, which are a source of fuel for our gut microbes.

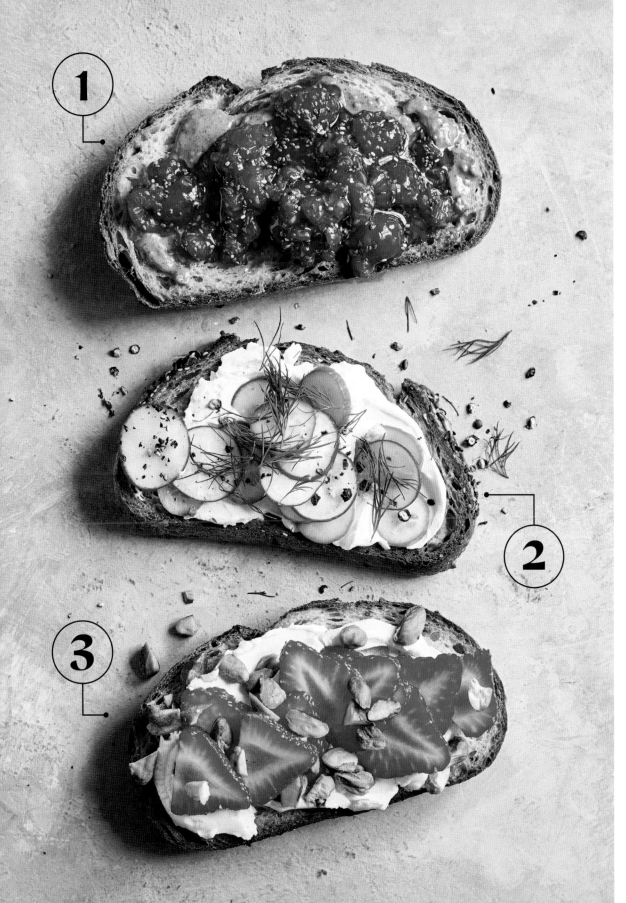

Sunshine Tomatoes + Labneh on Toast

SERVES 2

Plant Diversity
Score: 3
Bonus Score: 1.25

Labneh is a popular Middle Eastern probiotic soft cheese with a more complex flavour than yoghurt and a distinctive creamy tang. It is the perfect canvas for an array of toppings, from courgettes to smoked aubergines, olive oil and za'atar – even honey and walnuts for a sweet twist. This dish is a breakfast favourite of mine. Think of it like an Italian bruschetta that went on holiday to the Middle East, picking up some punchy flavours along the way.

—

4 large, thick slices
of sourdough bread

4 tsp extra-virgin olive oil,
plus a little extra for drizzling

1 garlic clove

200g (7oz) labneh
(or cream cheese)

180g (6oz) ripe cherry
tomatoes of various colours,
sliced in half

1 tbsp pomegranate molasses
(or balsamic vinegar)

½ tsp sumac

½ tsp dried oregano

½ tsp chilli flakes

Maldon sea salt

BONUS GUT-FRIENDLY TOPPINGS

Handful of finely chopped
parsley

Handful of pomegranate
seeds

1. Brush each slice of bread with a teaspoon of olive oil and toast in a hot griddle pan until charred and crisp. Rub the surface of each slice with the garlic clove, taking care not to squash the bread.

2. Spread the labneh over the slices of toast and top with the sliced tomatoes. Sprinkle over some sea salt. Drizzle the pomegranate molasses and more olive oil over the tomatoes, followed by a sprinkling of the sumac, oregano and chilli flakes. Top with chopped parsley and pomegranate seeds if you like.

the kitchen prescription

Tomato (Solanum lycopersicum)

+ Tomatoes are good for our eyes. They contain carotenoids such as lycopene $C_{40}H_{56}$ (which gives the red colour), lutein (which can help prevent cataracts) and beta-carotene (which benefits eye health).

+ Eating tomatoes with olive oil will assist in the absorption of carotenoids, so it is a good thing that tomatoes and olive oil taste so good together.

+ There is some evidence that tomato consumption may be associated with a lowered risk of developing prostate cancer and cardiovascular disease.

Five-Veg Masala Eggs

SERVES 4 GENEROUSLY

Plant Diversity
Score: 6

½ red onion, finely diced

2 spring onions, thinly sliced

1 tomato, finely chopped

½ yellow pepper, finely diced

½ leek, thinly sliced

6 free-range eggs

½ tsp ground turmeric

½ tsp red chilli powder

Handful of finely chopped coriander

1 tbsp olive oil

Salt, to taste

Plain omelettes can be replaced with this very satisfying combination of gently spiced eggs and vegetables. I often chop the vegetables the night before, so the next morning all you have to do is crack in the eggs. And any leftovers do very well in an omelette sandwich the next day. Use any vegetables you have to optimise your gut microbial diversity: peas, spinach, finely chopped green beans or broccoli would also make wonderful additions.

—

1. Place the red onion, spring onions, tomato, yellow pepper and leek in a bowl. Crack the eggs into the chopped vegetables and add the turmeric, chilli powder and coriander. Season with salt to taste and beat well.

2. Place a large non-stick frying pan over a medium heat and drizzle in the olive oil. When the pan is hot but not smoking, add the egg mixture. Tilt the pan slightly from side to side to allow the eggs to swirl and cover the surface of the pan completely.

3. When the mixture starts to set at the centre, scrape it with a spatula and tilt the pan again to allow the gaps to fill back up with the runny eggs. Repeat this process until the egg has just set: this takes about 2–3 minutes. At this point you can either attempt to flip the omelette whole or you can break it into quarters and flip each quarter to cook the top side till golden, this will take just another minute or so. Serve immediately.

Macatella

Plant Diversity
Score: 2.25
Bonus Score: 2

You've heard of Nutella, but what about Macatella? My take on the world's most famous nutty chocolate spread, Macatella is like Nutella but made with macadamia nuts. Why? Well, both macadamia nuts and good-quality cocoa are really good for your gut, so having this delicious gut-friendly spread with some warm toasted sourdough is going to be far better for you than slathering toast with shop-bought chocolatey spreads.

—

200g (7 oz) roasted macadamia nuts

4 tbsp icing sugar

100g (4oz) good-quality cocoa powder

Approximately 250ml (1 cup) kettle-hot water

Slices of toasted sourdough or other seedy wholegrain bread of your choice, to serve

Pinch of salt

BONUS GUT-FRIENDLY TOPPINGS

Chopped nuts or toasted seeds of your choice

Sliced banana or strawberries

1. Your macadamia nuts must be roasted here for the best flavour so if yours are not roasted, then put them into an oven preheated to 160°C fan/180°C/gas mark 4 for 12 minutes, or until they are golden. Allow to cool completely before use.

2. Start by blitzing the macadamia nuts, icing sugar and cocoa to as fine a powder as your food processor/blender will allow. (I use a NutriBullet or MagiMix for optimal smoothness.) Now add the majority of the hot water and blend again until you have a smooth spread with the approximate consistency of Nutella. If needed you can top up with more hot water. I find that the amount I use varies according to the quality of cocoa and nuts being used, so there is a bit of trial and error involved.

3. Store in a jar in the fridge for up to 2 weeks. Serve spread on toast, scattered with the salt. You can also add nuts or seeds and/or sliced banana or strawberries for a gut-friendly boost.

---

the kitchen prescription

Macadamia nuts (Macadamia integrifolia)

+ Like lots of other nuts that grow on trees, macadamia nuts contain compounds called tocotrienols, a type of vitamin E. These give protection to our nerve fibres, which is thought to protect an ageing brain.

+ Macadamia nuts are a rich source of heart-friendly monounsaturated fats. In fact, about 60 per cent of the whole kernel is made up of such fats.

+ Macadamia nuts are fibre-dense, which can help with staving off those hunger cravings for longer. They can also act as a prebiotic for your gut bugs.

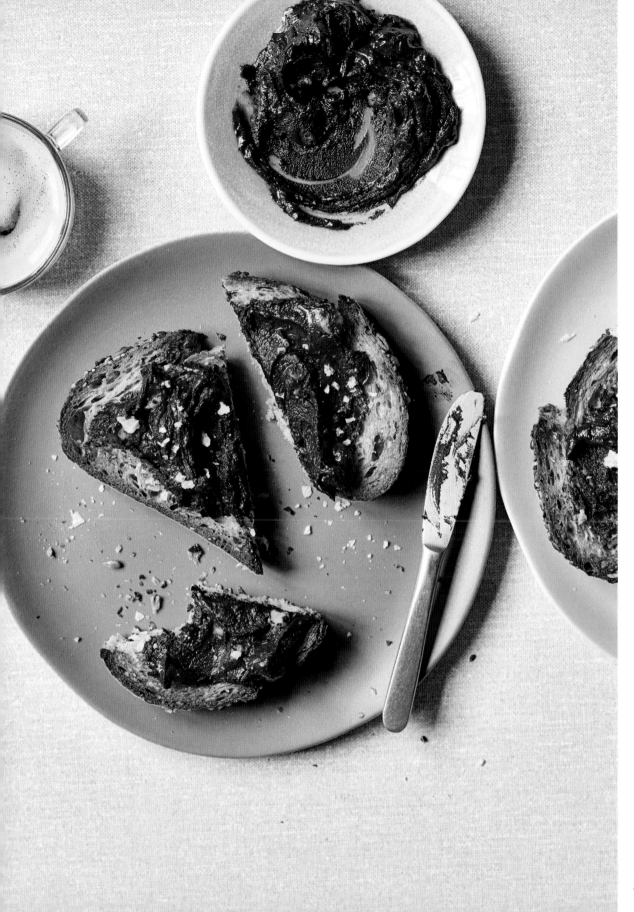

Ancient Grain Pancakes with Mascarpone, Hazelnuts + Date Molasses

MAKES 6–8

Plant Diversity
Score: 2.5
Bonus Score: 1 or more

75g (2¾oz/⅔ cup) khorasan flour (or wholewheat flour)

75g (2¾oz/⅔ cup) plain white flour

2 large free-range eggs

300ml (10fl oz/gnerous 1 cup) whole milk (or plant-based milk)

½ tsp ground turmeric

½ tsp ground cinnamon

1 tsp sugar

½ tsp salt

Vegetable oil, for cooking

TO SERVE

200g (7oz) mascarpone cheese or yoghurt (Greek or plant-based)

100g (3½oz) toasted hazelnuts, roughly chopped

Date molasses or maple syrup

BONUS GUT-FRIENDLY TOPPINGS

Chopped chunks of ripe banana, figs, chopped pitted dates or mango

Over thousands of years of cultivation, humans have developed numerous species of wheat through both natural selection and artificial selection by farmers. Khorasan is the common name for the ancient wheat grain Triticum turgidum. This gut-friendly, fibre-rich flour has a mild but nutty flavour, and its pale golden hue works incredibly well in these almost crêpe-like pancakes. Thankfully you can find it in most supermarkets nowadays, but if you can't, just use any wholewheat flour.

—

1. Mix both flours in a bowl with the eggs, milk, turmeric, cinnamon, sugar and salt. Whisk to combine well and ensure there are no lumps. The batter should be runny with the consistency of double cream. Allow the mixture to rest for 15 minutes.

2. Place a non-stick frying pan over a medium heat. Brush the pan with vegetable oil and pour in a ladleful of batter, swirling gently to spread the mix thinly. After a minute or two, flip the pancake and cook on the other side for the same time. You are aiming for a lacy, crêpe-like, golden brown pancake. Repeat with the remaining batter to make 6–8 pancakes.

3. Serve the pancakes with a spoonful of mascarpone, a sprinkling of hazelnuts and a generous drizzle of date molasses.

the kitchen prescription

Khorasan (Triticum turgidum ssp. turanicum)

+ Nutritional analysis of ancient khorasan wheat (known commercially as Kamut) versus modern wheat has found that it has a higher polyphenol content, giving it better antioxidant properties.

+ Dietary polyphenols support the growth of beneficial bacteria in the gut too. Khorasan boasts higher levels of copper, selenium and manganese than other wheat varieties.

+ Producers of the ancient grain claim that those people who feel they have an intolerance to gluten (but not a formal diagnosis of coeliac disease) often tolerate the grain better than common wheat; however, more research is needed to substantiate these claims. The grain contains gluten and should be avoided if you are diagnosed with coeliac disease.

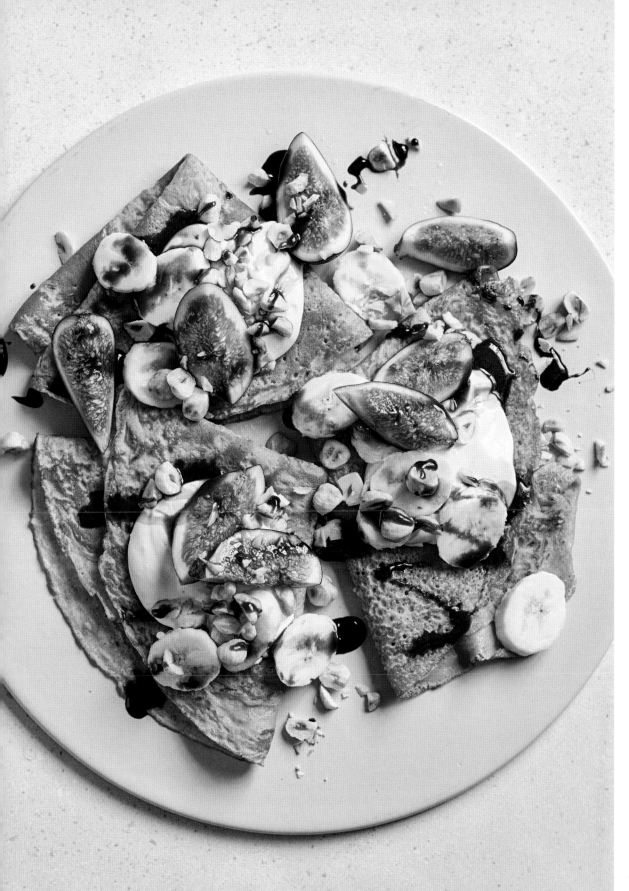

Breakfast Beans of Dreams

SERVES 4

Plant Diversity
Score: 3.75
Bonus Score: 1 or more

I grew up in the Middle East where this bean dish, called 'foul medammes', is a breakfast staple. Many cultures have their version of breakfast beans, whether it is baked beans on toast, Indian curried chickpeas with poori, or Mexican refried beans. It does make sense: beans are rich in gut microbe-fuelling fibre and protein, providing enough sustenance to stave hunger off until late in the afternoon. I use tinned fava beans here to save time, and you can often find these tins with 'foul medammes' written somewhere on the label. Use any other tinned beans such as kidney beans, chickpeas or black-eyed beans if you can't get hold of fava beans.

—

1 tbsp olive oil

2 garlic cloves, crushed

½ tsp cumin seeds

½ cinnamon stick

2 x 400g (14oz) tins fava beans

½ tsp hot paprika

½ tsp chilli flakes

300ml (10fl oz/generous 1 cup) kettle-hot water

Juice of ½ lemon

Salt, to taste

FOR THE RELISH

1 ripe tomato

2 tbsp olive oil

Handful of finely chopped parsley

TO SERVE

2 soft-boiled eggs

Selection of pickled vegetables, e.g. cucumbers, carrots and turnips

4 toasted pitta breads

1. Place the olive oil in a small saucepan over a low heat; when it has just started warming through, add the garlic, cumin seeds and cinnamon stick. The idea is to cook out the rawness of the garlic for a minute or two without letting it colour or burn.

2. Drain the fava beans and add them to the warm garlicky oil along with the paprika and chilli flakes. Top with the kettle-hot water and braise over a medium heat for about 20 minutes, stirring regularly. You will notice that the beans start breaking down slightly and thickening the whole mixture. Season with the lemon juice and salt to taste.

3. For the relish, grate the tomato into a small bowl. Add the olive oil and parsley and stir.

4. To serve, place the beans in individual small deep bowls. Top with the tomato relish and, if liked, half a soft-boiled egg. Pickled vegetables and toasted pitta breads are a fantastic side.

the kitchen prescription

Fava beans (Vicia faba L.)

+ Fava beans are legumes, which means they are a rich, inexpensive source of fibre and protein.

+ They are the prefect breakfast prebiotic, containing antioxidants and other bioactive compounds that are considered to contribute to human health.

+ Fava beans in particular are rich in folate, which supports the synthesis of DNA and is essential for the body to produce red blood cells.

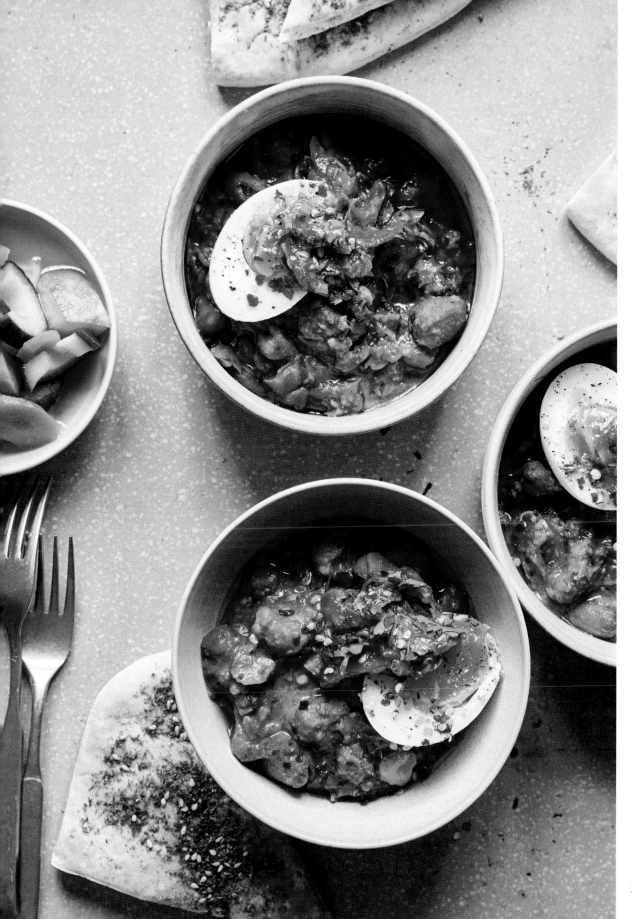

Poppy Seed Rösti with Smoked Salmon + Courgette Dill Crème

Plant Diversity
Score: 3.5

A classic example of how a breakfast dish can be made gut-friendly. Just a tablespoon of poppy seeds packs a massive 7g (¼oz) of gut-friendly fibre and adds a satisfying nutty crunch to the potato rösti base. Grating courgette (or indeed cucumber or beetroot) into the crème fraîche is a clever way of adding plant-based diversity to your diet. And last but not least, smoked salmon is packed full of omega-3 fatty acids, which are considered by many to exert a positive effect on intestinal microbiota. A feast for your taste buds and gut bugs in equal measure.

—

350g (12oz) waxy potatoes, grated (leave the skin on)

½ tsp flaky sea salt

1 level tbsp poppy seeds, plus a pinch to garnish

½ tsp dried oregano

1 tbsp cornflour

2 tbsp olive oil

150g (5oz) sliced smoked salmon

½ tsp crushed chilli flakes, to garnish

FOR THE COURGETTE DILL CRÈME

1 grated courgette (moisture squeezed out)

20g (¾oz) dill

20g (¾oz) chives

3 tbsp crème fraîche (or full-fat live Greek yoghurt)

½ tsp poppy seeds

Juice of ½–1 lemon

1. Place the grated potato in a piece of muslin or a clean J-cloth, gather the edges together and give the potatoes a really good squeeze to extract as much of the moisture as possible. (The drier your potatoes are, the crispier the rösti will be.) Place the potato in a bowl and add the salt, poppy seeds, oregano and cornflour. Stir well to combine.

2. Heat a large (about 30cm/12in in diameter) non-stick pan with a tablespoon of the olive oil over a medium heat. Tip in the potato mixture and gently press it down (carefully with your hands or with the back of a spoon). We are aiming for a disc that is about 25cm (10in) wide and 5mm (¼in) thick. Fry the rösti for about 8 minutes; you are looking for a really deep golden brown colour.

3. If you are looking at the rösti and fearing the dreaded flip, don't worry. Just use wooden board to cover the non-stick pan, then flip the board and pan together. Return the non-stick pan to the heat, drizzle in the remaining tablespoon of olive oil and slip the rösti from the board back into the pan. Fry for another 8 minutes or so till deeply golden. Gently slide the cooked rösti on to a serving platter.

4. To make the courgette crème, squeeze the moisture out of the grated courgette as you did for the potato. Tip this into a bowl with the dill, chives, crème fraîche/yoghurt, poppy seeds and lemon juice and mix together (keep a little of the dill and chives aside for garnishing). Top the rösti with the courgette crème mixture and then scatter over the slices of smoked salmon. Garnish with the remaining herbs, a touch of poppy seeds and the chilli flakes.

Charred Nectarines
with Yoghurt

Plant Diversity
Score: 1.25
Bonus Score: 1 or more

I enjoy this breakfast dish in the late summer months, when nectarines are sweet-fleshed and ripe, and the desire for a lighter, fresher breakfast prevails. I use Skyr, a popular Icelandic high-protein yoghurt, made by adding probiotic bacterial cultures to skimmed milk, then straining to remove the whey: it is almost made more like cheese than yoghurt. If nectarines are not in season, top the yoghurt with any fresh berries and nuts of your choice. Pistachios with strawberries or bananas with almonds are two of my other favourite gut-loving combinations.

—

4 nectarines, quartered and stoned (or use peaches)

1 tbsp maple syrup

6 mint leaves, thinly sliced into ribbons

450g (1lb) natural high-protein yoghurt, like Skyr

BONUS GUT-FRIENDLY TOPPINGS

1 tbsp toasted mixed seeds or 1 tbsp chopped pistachios, hazelnuts or almonds per portion

1. Place a griddle pan over a medium-high heat. When hot, add the nectarines, flesh side down, for 2 minutes. Turn them once and griddle the other side for about 2 minutes, or until char marks are visible on the fruit's surface. The idea is to soften the fruit and brings its juices to life, not to cook it completely.

2. Remove the nectarines from the griddle and place them in a serving dish. Dress the nectarines with maple syrup and strew delicately with the ribbons of mint. Top the yoghurt with the nectarines and serve immediately. Scatter over some toasted seeds or chopped nuts if you like.

BREAKFAST

LUNCH

Revitalise your midday⁺ meal

One of the things that I noticed after winning *MasterChef* was that work colleagues were suddenly terribly interested in the contents of my lunchbox. Each day they would examine my Tupperware trying to work out what slow-cooked aromatic delights it contained. Much of the time it housed delights like a bruised apple, random slices of cold pizza, or (if I was lucky) any food that one of my kids decided wasn't up to their required standard of service.

Now, I have zero qualms about taking leftovers from dinner to work with me. Sadly, in a household where both adults work, there are rarely enough leftovers for two. But whether it's him or me that gets to take the good stuff to work, it's a mathematical certainty that the other person will go without, instead having to make do with whatever the canteen, or more likely the vending machine, has available.

I realised that I should be doing more to prepare my lunches in advance. Here was a midday opportunity to optimise my gut health that I absolutely was not taking advantage of. Lunch is one of those things that to do well, you need to plan. It requires that extra bit of effort that few of us have the time, energy or motivation to expend. That is unless you want to end up spending a small fortune each day on some soggy sandwich and a bag of crisps.

To counteract this problem, I have developed a repertoire of quick and easy gut health-boosting sandwich and salad recipes that I can make the evening (or even a few days) before, laid out in batches ready for lunch. These make-ahead recipes make up the bulk of this chapter and you will find yourself coming back to them over and over again. There are also a few recipes for quick lunches you can rustle up in your lunchbreak at home, recognising that COVID-19 has changed many of our working patterns.

As you might expect, the recipes in this chapter are mostly plant-based. This is for two reasons: firstly, plant-based lunches are generally a bit quicker and cheaper to make than meat options, which often require a little longer on the cooker and are heavier on the wallet. Secondly, and arguably more importantly from this chef/doctor's point of view, these plant-focused recipes will help not just to feed you, but also to feed your inner community of beneficial gut microbes. The minimal effort and planning required to cook these dishes is, I hope you will agree, worth it to keep your gut in showroom-fresh condition.

Now that we've covered what to eat for lunch, we need to talk about how we should be eating our lunch. It's a sad reality that many of our workspaces and workplaces do not prioritise the lunchbreak. Many eat lunch in front of a computer screen checking emails, a hugely disadvantageous behaviour jeopardising both productivity and the opportunity to optimise gut health. Lunch should be a mindful moment where you chew food properly, to extract all nutrients and feed the body's appetite and gut bugs.

So, what are you waiting for? Get that gut of yours feeling good again with a solid, nutritious, and most importantly, consciously planned gut-loving lunch. And let's try to keep the absent-minded cold sandwiches at the desk, far, far away.

Chickpea Chilli Cheese Toastie

SERVES 2

Plant Diversity
Score: 4.5
Bonus Score: 1

If you work from home and want to try a gut-healthy protein- and fibre-packed version of a cheese toastie for lunch, look no further.
To add chilli heat I have used katta sambol paste, a Sri Lankan shallot and chilli paste which I buy online. You can substitute for a little caramelised onion chutney and some chilli, or use rose harissa or sriracha sauce instead.

—

1 x 400g (14oz) tin chickpeas, drained

1 heaped tsp katta sambol paste (or use one of the alternatives suggested above)

1 tbsp finely chopped coriander

1 spring onion, thinly sliced

50g (2oz/½ cup) grated mature Cheddar cheese

4 large slices of seeded sourdough bread

¼ red onion, thinly sliced

100g (3½oz/1 cup) grated mozzarella cheese

2 tbsp vegetable oil

BONUS GUT-FRIENDLY TOPPINGS

2 handfuls of baby spinach or watercress leaves

1. Combine the chickpeas in a bowl with the katta sambol paste, coriander, spring onion and Cheddar. Use the back of a fork to break the chickpeas down into a coarse paste. Spread the chickpea mixture over 2 of the slices of sourdough bread. Top the chickpeas with the red onion, followed by the mozzarella. Place the remaining 2 slices of bread on top to form 2 sandwiches ready to toast.

2. Place a large non-stick frying pan over a low heat. Brush both sides of each toastie with vegetable oil, then place them in the pan and press down with a weight (you may need to cook them one at a time). I use a flat plate weighed down with the lid of a cast-iron pot or tin of beans. Toast for about 5 minutes or so on each side until deeply golden and the cheese is oozing and melted. You can gently prise open the sandwich and stuff some spinach leaves inside if you wish. Serve immediately.

NOTE
You can make this recipe as a cold sandwich to take to work too. Just don't brush the surface of the bread with oil.

the kitchen prescription

Chickpeas (Cicer arietinum L.)

+ Chickpeas are great for your gut. The protein and fibre present in chickpeas is thought to increase the levels of appetite-reducing hormones in the body and increase the feeling of fullness. It's part of the reason why hummus is so filling.

+ Some small dietary intervention studies have suggested that

adding chickpeas to a predominantly wheat-based diet can significantly help reduce cholesterol levels.

+ Studies suggest that chickpeas can help you open the bowels more frequently and more easily compared to standard diets.

+ For more on chickpeas see page 124.

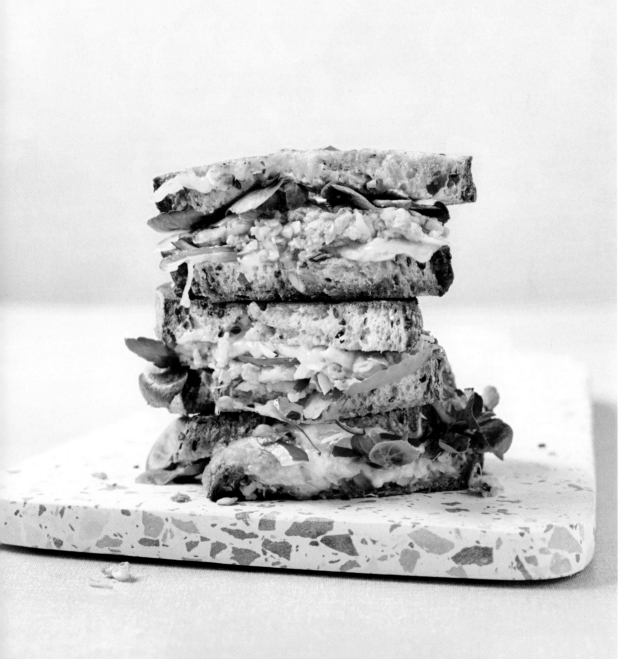

Arabian Nights Quinoa

SERVES 4

Plant Diversity
Score: 5.5
Bonus Score: 1.25

Quinoa is an excellent sponge for both flavour and moisture. I make this salad in batches at home. It lasts well in the fridge for a few days as the quinoa soaks up the watermelon and cucumber juice. I often take a few mint leaves and nuts with me to work in a separate pot and strew them over the salad before greedily devouring... much to the envy of all around me.

—

125g (4oz) dried tricolour quinoa

½–1 red chilli, thinly sliced

Juice of 1–2 limes

2 tsp rosewater

2 tsp honey

2 tbsp olive oil

300g (10oz) watermelon, cut into 3cm (1¼in) cubes

200g (7oz) cucumber, deseeded and sliced into half-moons

100g (3½oz) vegetarian feta cubes

Salt, to taste

TO FINISH

2 tbsp nuts of your choice, e.g. flaked almonds or pistachios

Handful of whole mint leaves

1. Cook the quinoa in boiling water according to the packet instructions. Drain and set aside.

2. Combine the red chilli, lime juice, rosewater, honey and olive oil in a small bowl. Mix well to form a dressing.

3. Toss the quinoa, watermelon, cucumber and feta together and drizzle over the dressing, then mix gently to combine. Season with salt to taste, then divide between 4 Tupperware boxes and refrigerate until ready to eat. Scatter over the nuts and mint leaves just before eating.

---

the kitchen prescription

Quinoa (Chenopodium quinoa)

+ Though technically (botanically) speaking a seed, quinoa is classified as a whole grain.

+ It is gluten free and comes in black, red, yellow and white varieties.

+ As a general rule, the darker the quinoa, the higher its antioxidant capacity.

+ Red and black quinoa contain almost double the vitamin E content compared to white quinoa. Vitamin E acts as an antioxidant, scavenging loose electrons called free radicals that can damage cells. It maintains healthy skin and eyes and strengthens the body's natural defence against illness and infection.

+ Quinoa is a complete protein, which means that it contains all nine essential amino acids (see page 16).

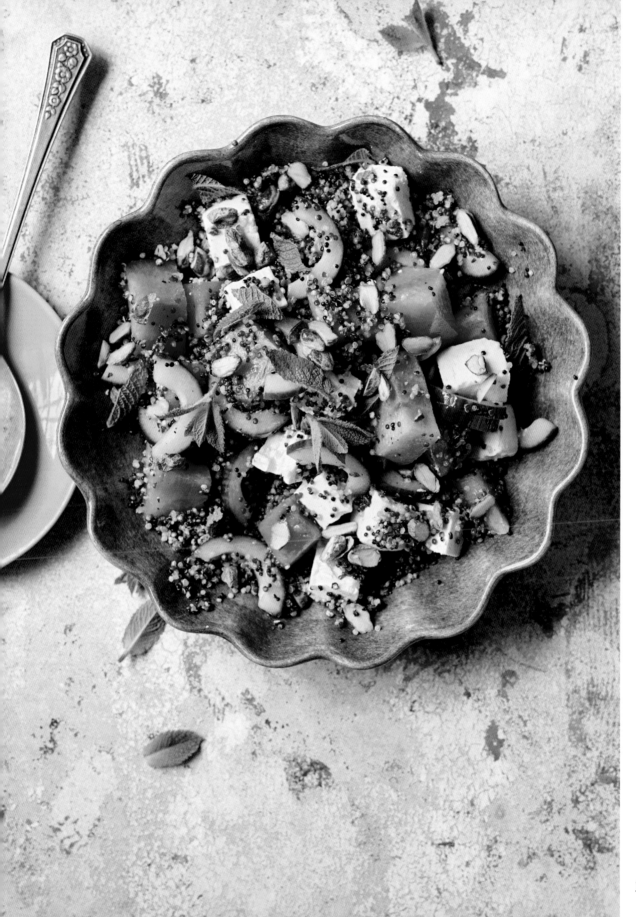

Egg + Sauerkraut Mayo on Rye

SERVES 1

Plant Diversity
Score: 3.5

Rye bread is a fibre-dense, heavy loaf, made with very few ingredients and sliced into thin rectangles. It is rich in bioactive lignans, which are plant compounds thought to be responsible for reducing our risk of heart disease, stroke and even menopausal symptoms, so it's well worth developing a taste for. I take these rye bread sandwiches to work on days where I am working late shifts; they keep me full late into the evening.

—

2 hard-boiled eggs

2 tbsp sauerkraut (see Note)

1 tbsp mayonnaise

½ tsp caraway seeds

Large handful of watercress

1 tsp olive oil

2 rectangular slices of Polish rye and sunflower seed bread

1. Peel the eggs and slice them into quarters. Combine the sauerkraut with the mayonnaise and caraway seeds. Dress the watercress with olive oil.

2. To assemble the sandwich, take one slice of bread as the base. Spoon over the sauerkraut mayo and then layer over the egg quarters. Strew the watercress over the eggs before placing the other slice of rye bread over the top. Slice in half with a sharp knife and pack in clingfilm or foil to transport to work. Alternatively, just eat there and then!

NOTE
To make your own sauerkraut, shred 2kg (4½lb) cabbage into a large mixing bowl and rub 5 teaspoons of flaky sea salt into it with clean hands for about 5 minutes (or until there is quite a bit of moisture at the bottom of the bowl). Add spices of your choice at this point and pack the cabbage and its briny juices into sterilised jars, ensuring that the liquid rises high enough to cover the kraut (top up with filtered water if necessary). Leave 2.5cm (1in) at the top of the jar empty for expansion. Leave it to ferment naturally for a few days, opening the jar to release the gas daily before transferring to the fridge.

the kitchen prescription

Sauerkraut

+ Sauerkraut is made from shredded raw cabbage fermented in brine by lactic acid bacteria.

+ It is a probiotic and is thought to exert a beneficial effect on our gut microbiota. While the studies looking at the health benefits of sauerkraut are fairly limited,

early work points to benefits for the immune system and inflammation.

+ Probiotic effects aside, I would encourage you try it on the grounds that it tastes wonderful. It goes particularly well with sausages, dill, apple and mustard.

Spiced Potato Salad with Tomatoes + Broad Beans

SERVES 2-4

Plant Diversity
Score: 5
Bonus Score: 2

This potato salad is a wonderful lunchbox treat inspired by the street food of India. Surprised to see a recipe featuring potato in a gut health cookbook? One of the most common questions people ask me is whether carbohydrates (such as potatoes) are bad for their gut. The answer is that we need carbohydrates as part of a balanced diet. But not all carbs are not created equal; there is a vast difference between the carbohydrates in bulgur wheat versus the refined carbohydrates in sausage roll pastry. The trick is to include good, natural sources of carbohydrates in your diet while minimising the refined stuff where possible.

—

500g (1lb 2oz) boiled
new potatoes, skin on

150g (5oz) blanched
broad beans

2 ripe tomatoes, halved and
thinly sliced

1 tbsp olive oil

½ tsp red chilli powder

1 tsp chaat masala

½ tsp toasted cumin seeds

2 tbsp finely chopped
coriander

Juice of ½ lemon

Salt, to taste

**FOR THE GREEN CASHEW
CHUTNEY (OPTIONAL)**

125g (4oz/1 cup) cashews

125g (4oz/¾ cup) golden
sultanas

60g (2½oz) roughly chopped
coriander

75ml (5 tbsp/⅓ cup) lemon
juice

1 green chilli

Salt, to taste

1. Quarter the new potatoes and add to a bowl with all the remaining ingredients. Toss everything together gently to ensure that the spices coat all the potatoes evenly.

2. To make the green chutney, blend all the ingredients together with a splash of water (I do this in a nutribullet).

3. Serve the potato salad with the chutney alongside – this tastes best served at room temperature.

LUNCH

---

the kitchen prescription

Potatoes (Solanum tuberosum)

+ Get the most out of your potatoes by cooking them in their skins – and eating the skins too.

+ When you cook and cool potatoes, the starch granules become 'resistant starches' that cannot be broken down as easily our stomach enzymes. This means that you won't experience the quick spike in blood sugars that can leave you feeling lethargic.

+ The reason resistant starches are useful is that a more gradual rise and fall in blood sugar levels (and therefore a more measured, steady release of insulin) is useful for healthy weight management. You can cook and cool other starches such as rice and pasta to increase the ratio of resistant starch in your meal.

Gut Glory Wraps

SERVES 1

Plant Diversity Scores:
5.25; 6; 4; 6.25; 4

Fill wholewheat wraps with a range of diverse fillings that feed your inner community. I have offered five different wrap filling options here, so you can try a different one for every day of the week if you wish! It's worth bearing in mind that there are a number of recipes that feature across *The Kitchen Prescription* that would make fabulous wrap fillings – see Vibrant Green Paneer (page 150), Limey Pickle Roast Cauliflower Popcorn (page 204) or Turkish Carrots in Saffron Sauce (page 193).

1. Goats' Cheese, Pea + Mint Wraps

1 tbsp hummus
2 heaped tbsp defrosted peas
100g (3½oz) drained tinned green lentils
60g (2½oz) crumbled goats' cheese
8 mint leaves
Handful of spinach leaves

Spread the hummus across the wrap. Gently crush the peas, lentils and cheese with a fork and layer on to the hummus. Top with the mint and spinach, roll tightly and wrap in foil, paper or clingfilm.

2. Cannellini Bean, Pesto, Avocado + Spinach Wraps

1 heaped tbsp pesto
100g (3½oz) drained tinned cannellini beans
½ avocado, chopped into rough chunks
3 cherry tomatoes, halved
Handful of spinach leaves

Spread the pesto over the base of the wrap and top with the beans, avocado and tomatoes. Layer on the spinach leaves. Roll tightly and wrap in foil, paper or clingfilm.

3. Beetroot, Cottage Cheese + Walnut Wraps

75g (2¾oz) grated beetroot
2 tbsp cottage cheese
Handful of spinach leaves
6 roughly chopped walnuts

Squeeze the moisture out of the grated beetroot, then combine with the cottage cheese. Layer the spinach leaves on the bottom of the wrap, top with the cottage cheese and beetroot mixture, followed by the walnuts. Roll tightly and wrap in foil, paper or clingfilm.

4. Rainbow Rolls

2 tbsp hummus
½ grated carrot
½ red pepper, thinly sliced
Handful of thinly sliced red cabbage
3 jarred artichokes, roughly chopped
Handful of roughly chopped parsley
Squeeze of lemon juice

Spread the hummus over the base of your wrap before loading with all the vegetables, parsley and lemon juice. Roll tightly and wrap in foil, paper or clingfilm.

5. Tandoori Chicken + Mango Chutney Wraps

1 tbsp mayonnaise
1 tsp tandoori masala
100g (3½oz) leftover cooked chicken
¼ cucumber, deseeded and sliced into half-moons
1 tbsp mango chutney
Handful of watercress leaves

Mix the mayonnaise with the tandoori masala and leftover chicken in a small bowl. Lay the dressed chicken on the wrap, then top with cucumber, mango chutney and watercress leaves. Roll tightly and wrap in foil, paper or clingfilm.

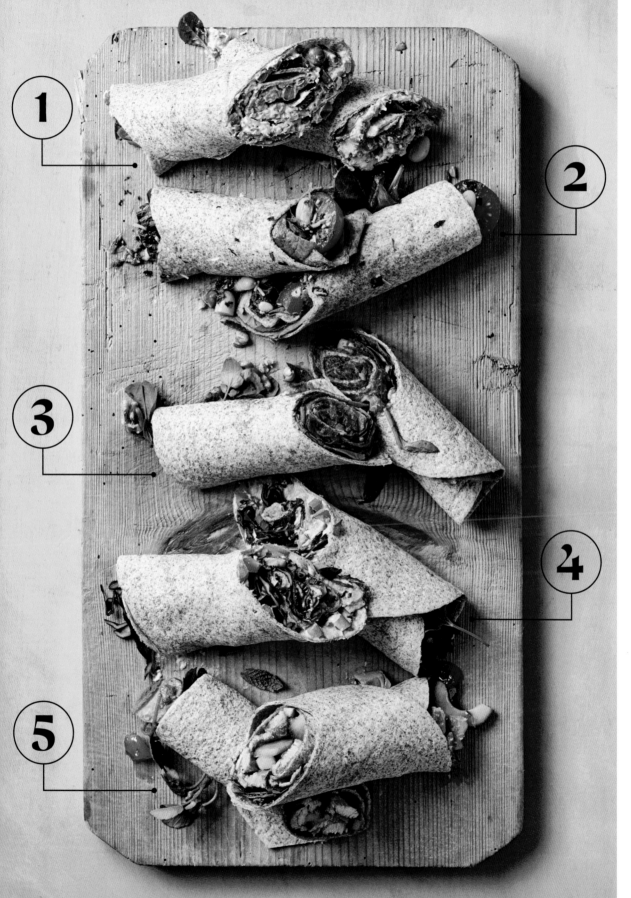

Mackerel Salad Sandwiches

SERVES 2

Plant Diversity
Score: 4

On the banks of the Bosphorus river in Istanbul at lunchtime you find roadside carts selling chargrilled fresh mackerel salad sandwiches called *balik ekmek*. Mackerel has a wonderful, rich flavour, is micronutrient-dense and often comes ready to eat. For some reason it is constantly overlooked by people doing their weekly shops; this flavour-packed recipe will hopefully go some way towards changing this.

—

2 fillets of vacuum-packed smoked mackerel (100g/3½oz each)

2 slices of French baguette, about 15cm/6in long each

FOR THE SALAD

75g (2¾oz) grated carrot

¼ red onion, thinly sliced

1 ripe tomato, halved then thinly sliced

Handful of roughly chopped parsley

FOR THE SALAD DRESSING

1 tbsp olive oil

Juice ½ lemon

1 tsp honey

1 tsp pomegranate molasses (or balsamic vinegar)

½ tsp chilli flakes

½ tsp garlic granules

½ tsp sumac (optional)

1. Start by heating a non-stick pan over a medium heat. Place the mackerel fillets (keep the skin on) in the non-stick pan and crisp them up by cooking for 2 minutes on each side. Mackerel is a very oily fish and as it cooks will release lots of oil into the pan, so no extra oil is needed.

2. Carefully remove the mackerel and place and on a plate. Slice your baguettes in half and place them face down in the non-stick pan. The baguettes will soak up the oily mackerel juices and crisp up in just a few minutes.

3. Mix all the ingredients for the salad dressing in a bowl and whisk well to combine. Pour this dressing over the carrots, onion, tomato and parsley.

4. To serve, place the salad at the base of the toasted baguette and top with the crispy mackerel fillet, followed by the lid of the baguette. Serve immediately or pack for lunch.

the kitchen prescription

Mackerel

+ Mackerel is considered by many to be a key component of a cardio-protective diet and is recognised as a crucial contributor to a healthier metabolic profile.

+ Being an oily fish, mackerel is a fantastic source of omega-3 oils (which our gut bugs love).

+ Mackerel is a source of vitamin B12 and has variable (but impressive) vitamin D content.

+ Mackerel is naturally abundant in selenium, an important chemical that supports healthy immunity and brain function.

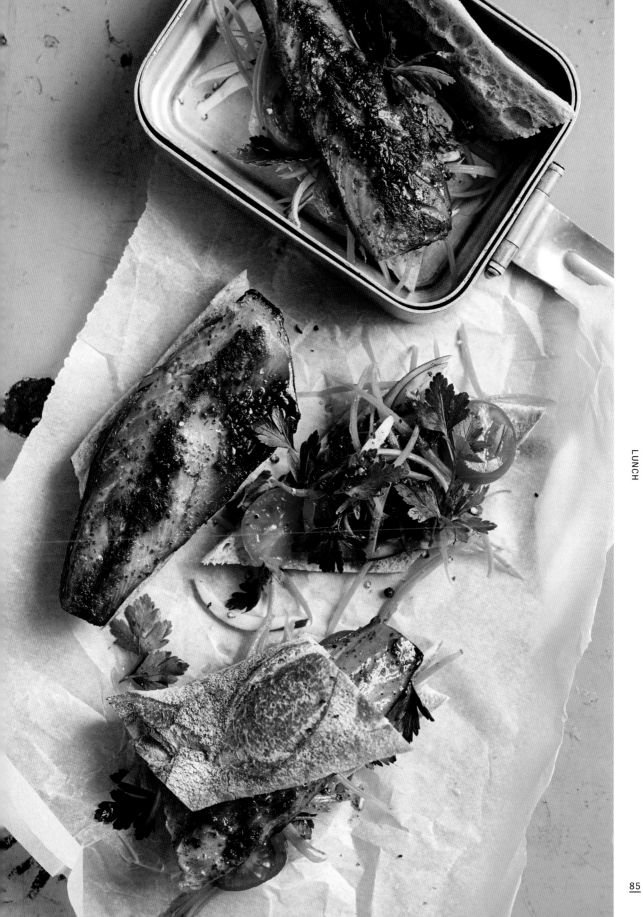

Ruby Red Polyphenol Salad

SERVES 4

Plant Diversity
Score: 5.25

This colourful fruit and vegetable salad is packed to the brim with plant polyphenols. Polyphenols are not just antioxidants, protecting our bodies' cells from damage and chronic inflammation, they also interact and help modulate our intestinal microbes for the better. So it's well worth having this tutti-frutti vegetable delight lurking in the fridge.

—

½ small red cabbage, thinly sliced

1 red apple, cored and finely chopped

1 red onion, thinly sliced

300g (10oz) red seedless grapes, halved

300g (10oz) pomegranate seeds

Juice of 1 lemon

300ml (10fl oz/generous 1 cup) crème fraîche or soured cream

½–1 tsp chilli flakes

Salt, to taste

1. Combine the cabbage, apple, red onion, grapes and pomegranate seeds in a mixing bowl. Add the lemon juice, crème fraîche, chilli flakes and salt to taste. Mix everything well and divide between 4 Tupperware boxes before transferring to the fridge.

2. The purplish colours will intensify as the salad sits in the fridge; I feel it tastes even better after 24–48 hours of resting.

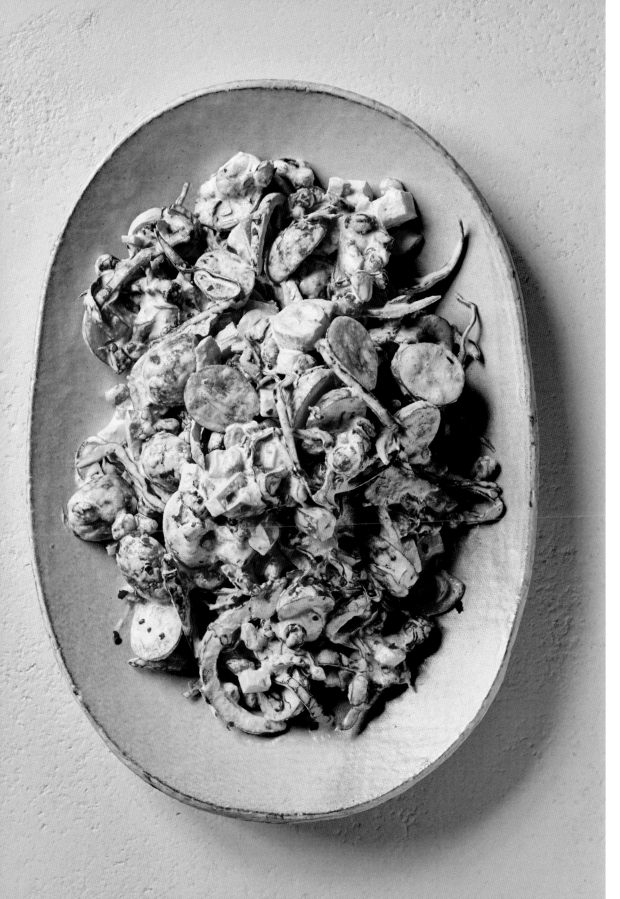

Kimchi + Pineapple Virtue Bowls

MAKES 2

Plant Diversity
Score: 8

Virtue bowls are an easily transportable lunch option and are open to endless adaptation depending on your taste preferences and what you have to hand. This is how I design a customised gut-friendly virtue bowl:

+ Start with a starch. I use wholegrain rice or brown rice, but you can use cooked and cooled sushi rice, which is high in resistant starches and prevents big surges in blood sugar. You can basically use any leftover cooked grain.

+ Try to include at least 2–3 vegetables or fruits. Finely diced peppers, avocado chunks, grated carrots, steamed broccoli or cauliflower, radishes, peas, edamame beans, pineapple and mango chunks work really well.

+ Include a handful of protein such as prawns, salmon, tuna or leftover chicken. For a vegan option, add some nice firm chunks of tofu or tempeh.

+ Finish the virtue bowl with a probiotic fermented condiment, for example kimchi or sauerkraut.

—

200g (7oz) cooked wholegrain rice

75g (2¾oz) grated carrots

¼ cucumber, deseeded and sliced into half-moons

100g (3½oz) edamame beans

150g (5oz) diced pineapple

150g (5oz) kimchi

150g (5oz) cooked jumbo prawns

2 tsp crispy fried onions

1 tsp black sesame seed seeds

FOR THE DRESSING

2 tsp sesame oil

2 tsp honey

4 tsp rice vinegar

1–2 red chillies, finely chopped

2 tbsp finely chopped coriander

2 tbsp water

1. Divide the rice, carrot, cucumber, edamame beans, pineapple, kimchi and prawns equally between 2 shallow bowls. Sprinkle the crispy fried onions over the rice and the sesame seeds over the pineapple chunks or carrots.

2. Mix the sesame oil, honey, rice vinegar, red chilli, coriander and water together in a small bowl to form a dressing to serve alongside the final dish. If you are taking the dish for lunch, transport the dressing in a separate small Tupperware box and pour over your bowl just before eating.

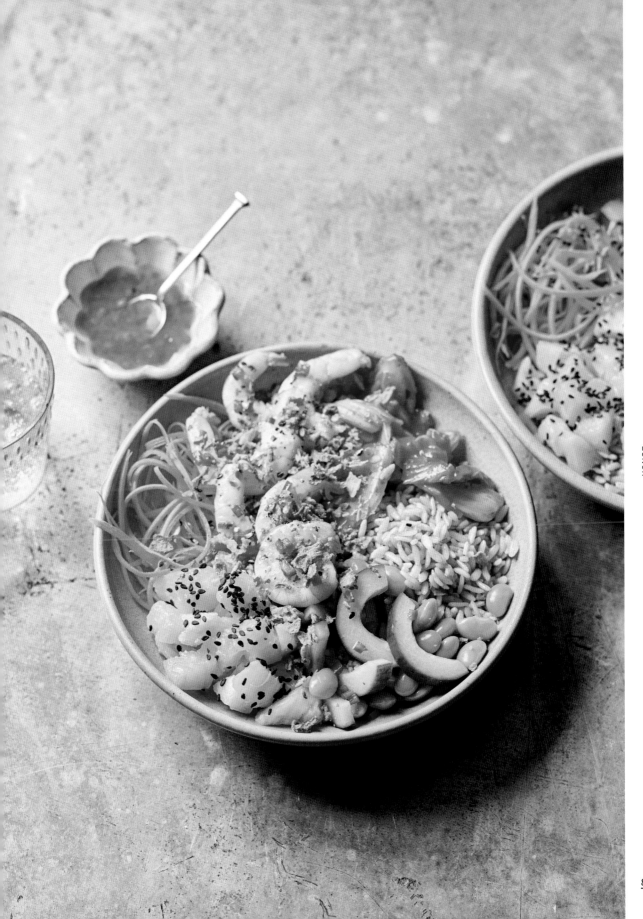

Green Gut Goddess Salad

SERVES 4-6

```
Plant Diversity
Score: 8
```

The 'Green Goddess' salad has enjoyed much popularity on TikTok. My version is packed full of extra gut-healthy, prebiotic cruciferous vegetables such as cabbage, broccoli and kale, all designed to boost gut microbial diversity. It keeps well, like coleslaw would, and can be enjoyed with tortilla chips or other crispbreads. The key is to take time to chop the vegetables finely before tossing them in the vivid green dressing.

—

200g (7oz) Tenderstem broccoli

½ small green cabbage, finely diced

½ cucumber, deseeded and diced into small cubes

4 spring onions, thinly sliced

50g (2oz) kale, finely shredded (remove tough stems first)

FOR THE DRESSING

Juice of 2 large lemons

50g (2oz) baby spinach

20g (¾oz) basil leaves

20g (¾oz) chives

2 garlic cloves

1 tbsp maple syrup

100ml (3½fl oz/scant ½ cup) extra-virgin olive oil

100g (3½oz/¾ cup) cashews

2 tbsp nutritional yeast

1. Bring a saucepan of water to the boil, add the broccoli and blanch for just 30 seconds, then drain and run under cold water. Finely chop the broccoli, then add to a large mixing bowl with all the other chopped vegetables.

2. Blend all the ingredients for the dressing together in a blender or nutribullet until very smooth.

3. Pour the dressing over the chopped vegetables and mix well to combine. Divide between Tupperware boxes and refrigerate until you are ready for lunch.

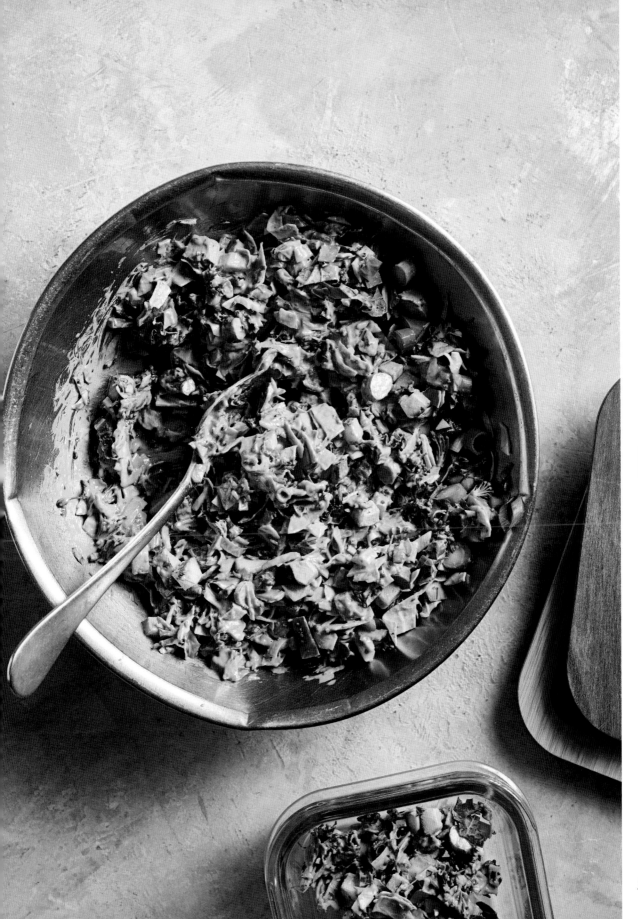

Spelt with Beetroot, Blue Cheese, Walnut + Dill

SERVES 4

Plant Diversity
Score: 3.5
Bonus Score: 1

This lunchbox dish is an entire lesson on how to feed your gut microbiome. The prebiotic fibre-dense wholegrain spelt is dyed purple with polyphenol-rich beetroot, only to then be bathed in a probiotic live yoghurt, and finally flecked with live probiotic blue cheese and a spattering of herbs and nuts. There is also room for flexibility in this dish; for example, if you are not a fan of blue cheese, then simply omit it. You can also use any other grain of your choice, like pearl barley or bulgur wheat.

—

200g (7oz/1 cup) dried pearl spelt

300g (10oz) steamed and ready-to-eat vacuum-packed beetroot

3 tbsp live natural yoghurt

20g (¾oz) fresh dill, finely chopped, plus a few sprigs to garnish

Juice of 1 lemon

1 tbsp extra-virgin olive oil

Handful of roughly chopped toasted walnuts

100g (3½oz) blue cheese, e.g. Gorgonzola or Cashel blue

Salt and black pepper, to taste

BONUS GUT-FRIENDLY ADDITIONS

For extra plant diversity and textural contrast, add a finely chopped Granny Smith apple

1. Prepare the dried spelt according to the packet instructions. It usually needs to be boiled for just under 30 minutes, or until tender. Drain and set aside.

2. Roughly chop the beetroot into small chunks and place them in a bowl. Mix the spelt with the beetroot, then add the yoghurt, dill, lemon juice and olive oil. Season with about 15 twists of the pepper mill and add salt to taste.

3. To serve the spelt, toss over the walnuts and a few flecks of blue cheese. Finish with a few sprigs of extra dill if you have some. This keeps very well in the fridge for 2–3 days – the longer you keep it, the more intense the colour will become. Add a finely chopped apple for a extra plant diversity.

---

the kitchen prescription

Beetroot (Beta vulgaris L.)

+ Beetroots are a complex mix of multiple biologically active phytochemicals, including betalains, flavonoids, polyphenols and saponins.

+ Many very robust studies seem to suggest that beetroot has cardioprotective qualities,

in that it may lower blood pressure.

+ Beetroot is also thought to exert a positive response on blood sugar and therefore may have a role in preventing diabetes.

Orzo with Pepper, Chilli + Orange

SERVES 4

```
Plant Diversity
Score: 5
Bonus Score: 2
```

Orzo has long been a used in pasta salads; this combination with peppers, chilli and orange is properly irresistible. Add any other vegetables or one of the gut-friendly additions to boost gut microbial diversity still further. Make this dish and divide into four Tupperware boxes (once thoroughly cooled) for a delicious, gut-healthy, make-ahead lunch.

—

6 red and yellow peppers, halved and deseeded

4 tbsp olive oil

3 large oranges

250g (9oz/1¼ cups) dried orzo

1 tbsp tomato purée

1 tbsp red chilli paste

Juice of 1 lemon

1 tsp sumac

50g (2oz) parsley, chopped

Salt, to taste

```
BONUS GUT-FRIENDLY
ADDITIONS
```

Handful of chopped roasted hazelnuts

Handful of pomegranate seeds

1. Preheat the oven to 180°C fan/200°C/gas mark 6. Place the peppers on a baking sheet, drizzle over 2 tablespoons of the olive oil and season liberally with salt. Transfer to the oven and roast for about 30 minutes until the peppers are completely softened and charred at the edges. Remove from the oven and set aside to cool. Once cool, slice the peppers into thin slices. (You can skip this stage and buy shop-bought roasted peppers in a jar if you prefer.)

2. Slice off the top and bottom of each orange. Next, use even, downward strokes to slice the peel away and white pith from the flesh. Discard the peel. Now cut between the membranes to segment the pieces of orange flesh.

3. Cook the orzo in well salted boiling water according to the packet instructions (this usually takes about 5 minutes). Drain the pasta, reserving the pasta water.

4. Heat the remaining olive oil in large pan over a medium heat. Add the tomato purée and chilli paste, followed by the lemon juice and sumac. Tumble in the drained orzo along with the roasted peppers and a good glug of leftover pasta water. Give everything a thorough mix and heat through; it will be ready within the next minute or two. Taste the dish and add some salt if you feel it needs more.

5. Allow to cool slightly, then top the orzo with parsley and the segmented oranges before serving. Scatter over hazelnuts and pomegranate seeds if desired.

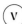

Chipotle Chilli Wild Rice

SERVES 2

Plant Diversity
Score: 4.75
Bonus Score: 2

It's rumoured that when footballer Romelu Lukaku moved from Manchester United to Inter Milan, a nutritionist was brought in to help him lose weight and to get him into the best physical shape of his life. Apparently, his new diet included a hefty amount of wild rice! If it is good enough for the gut of an athlete that Inter Milan paid 80 million euros for, then its good enough for mine too. Double or triple the quantities and leave out the coriander if you are preparing a large batch to take to work over the next few days – simply scatter fresh coriander and avocado on before eating. This keeps very well in the fridge and can be eaten hot or cold.

—

250g (9oz) cooked wild rice (use ready-cooked packs for ease)

½ red onion, thinly sliced

1 x 200g (7oz) tin sweetcorn (drained weight 165g/6oz)

100g (3½oz) jarred charred red peppers, thinly sliced

2 tbsp olive oil

Juice of 1 lime

1–2 tsp chipotle chilli paste

2 tbsp finely chopped coriander

Salt, to taste

BONUS GUT-FRIENDLY ADDITIONS

1 avocado, sliced into thin slices/small chunks

Handful of halved cherry tomatoes

1. Place the cooked rice, red onion, sweetcorn and peppers in a small bowl.

2. In another bowl, mix together the olive oil, lime juice and chipotle chilli paste and season with salt to taste. You can use more or less of the chipotle paste depending on your preference and how strong the paste you have to hand is.

3. Pour this dressing over the rice and vegetable mix and toss everything together to combine well. Top with chopped coriander and avocado and/or cherry tomatoes just before serving.

the kitchen prescription

Wild rice (Zizania palustris, aquatica, texana and latifolia)

+ Surprisingly, wild rice is technically not actually rice. It is the seed of an aquatic grass (like rice) but isn't directly related to it.

+ It grows abundantly in shallow freshwater marshes, along the shores of lakes. Three of the four wild rice species are native to North America, while the fourth is native to Asia.

+ Wild rice boasts impressive amounts of several nutrients, including protein. Wild rice is a complete protein, which means it contains all nine essential amino acids that our body cannot produce on its own and which are needed to build protein in our bodies. Therefore, wild rice is good to include in your diet if you are building muscle or are vegan or vegetarian.

+ The fibre content is similar to brown rice but it possesses about 30 per cent fewer calories than brown rice and significantly more protein.

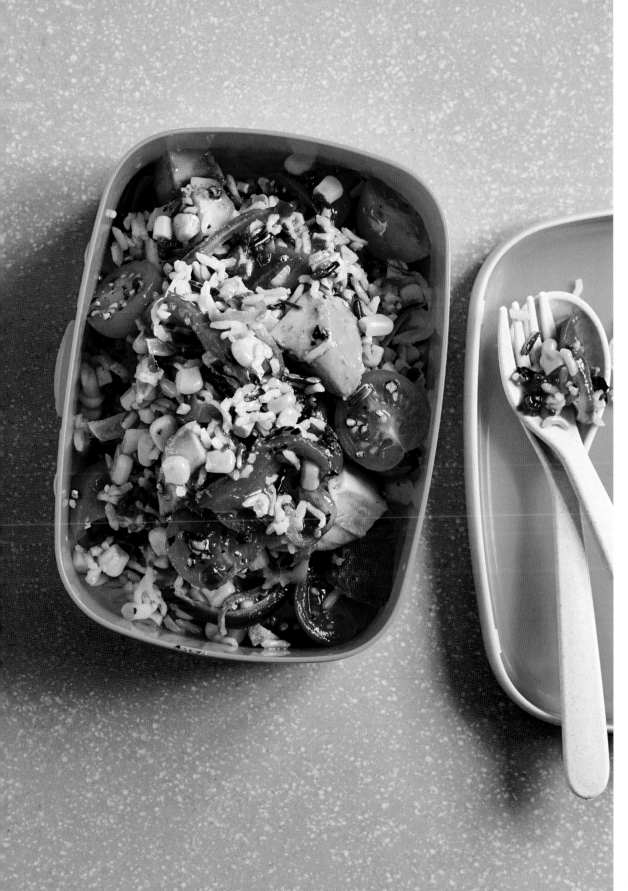

'Kimcheese' Frittata

SERVES 4

Plant Diversity
Score: 3

Very few lunch items fill me with joy as much as a frittata. If you are working from home you can enjoy it straight from the grill. Alternatively, make it the night before, allow it to cool, then cut into thick wedges for your lunchbox. I like to serve it alongside some fresh kimchi; the combination of fresh and cooked cabbage works wonders for the taste buds and the gut microbes.

—

3 large free-range eggs

2 heaped tbsp plain flour

6 spring onions, finely chopped

160g (5½oz) kimchi, roughly chopped, extra juice discarded, plus extra to serve

125g (4oz/1¼ cups) grated mature Cheddar cheese

1 generous tbsp vegetable oil

1 heaped tsp black sesame seeds

Salt, to taste

1. Preheat your grill to its highest setting. Beat the eggs and plain flour together to form a batter-like mixture. Add the spring onions, kimchi and all but a generous handful of the cheese to the batter. Season with a touch of salt and beat everything well to combine.

2. Heat a tablespoon of vegetable oil in a small non-stick pan until hot, but not smoking. Pour in the frittata batter and cook over a medium heat for 3 or so minutes. Scatter over the remaining cheese and sprinkle over the sesame seeds before sliding under the grill for another 3–4 minutes, or until the cheese is bubbly and golden. Remove from the grill very carefully as the handle may be very hot.

3. You can leave the frittata in the pan or allow it to cool slightly before sliding it out on to a board. Serve alongside some more fresh kimchi.

NOTE
For extra plant diversity add whatever vegetables to your frittata that you have in your kitchen which you think might work. I like to add grated carrots and sweetcorn, but experiment with what works for you.

the kitchen prescription

Kimchi

+ In this Korean speciality, Chinese cabbage is salted and then seasoned with a variety of spices including Korean red pepper powder, garlic and ginger, before being fermented with a mixture of lactic acid bacteria in a process known as lacto-fermentation.

+ Kimchi is considered a probiotic. Some provisional studies have shown that while contributing to gut microbial diversity and weight management, it can also stimulate our immune systems.

+ Korean adults consume an estimated 100g (3½oz) of kimchi a day! Some scientists believe that this in part may be responsible for the long life expectancy of the Korean population.

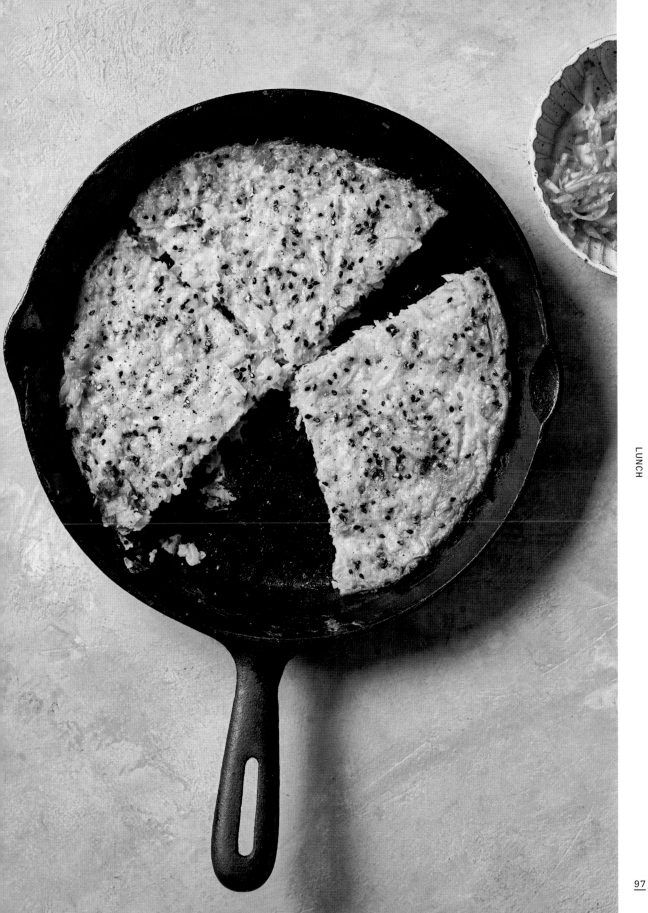

Gut Love Pot Noodles

Plant Diversity
Score: 6.25

We all have our weaknesses, and mine is a pot noodle. These noodles are just as satisfying as the shop-bought variety, but so much better for your gut. As with many others in this chapter, this recipe is for guidance and can be adapted to your preferences. All you need to get started is a large jar.

—

120g (4oz) cooked udon or other noodles tossed in 1 tsp vegetable oil

50g (2oz) mangetout, thinly sliced

30g (1oz) edamame beans

¼ carrot, grated

2 baby sweetcorn, sliced in half lengthways

1 spring onion, finely diced

1 heaped tsp crunchy peanut butter

½–1 tsp miso paste

1 heaped tsp chilli oil

1. Layer a jam jar with the noodles, mangetout, edamame beans, carrot, baby sweetcorn and spring onion.

2. Combine the peanut butter, miso paste and chilli oil in a small bowl. Pour this dressing over the layered vegetables and noodles and screw the jam jar lid on. Place in the fridge until ready to use.

3. When you are ready to eat the noodles, pour just enough boiling water from a kettle to cover the noodles. Allow to sit for a few minutes before stirring well and serving.

4. I eat directly from the jam jar, but you can decant into a deep serving bowl if you prefer. If you like your vegetables a little more cooked, you can place the jam jar full of noodles, vegetables and water (but without the lid) in the microwave for a minute or two so that the vegetables are no longer al dente.

the kitchen prescription

Noodles

+ Shirataki noodles, otherwise known as konjac yam or miracle noodles are made by mixing glucomannan flour with lime water. Glucomannan is a very viscous soluble fibre that absorbs water to form a gel. It is thought to promote feelings of fullness and lead to weight loss.

+ Soba noodles are an incredibly versatile and delicious nutty noodle made from 100 per cent buckwheat flour. They are very popular in Japanese cuisine

and rich in protein, gut-friendly soluble fibre and microminerals like manganese and thiamine. Buckwheat flour, despite its name, is actually gluten free.

+ You can make your own gut-friendly noodles at home using ancient grain flour like khorasan (Kamut) and egg. Simply knead well, rest the mixture for a short time, then roll and cut into thin strips.

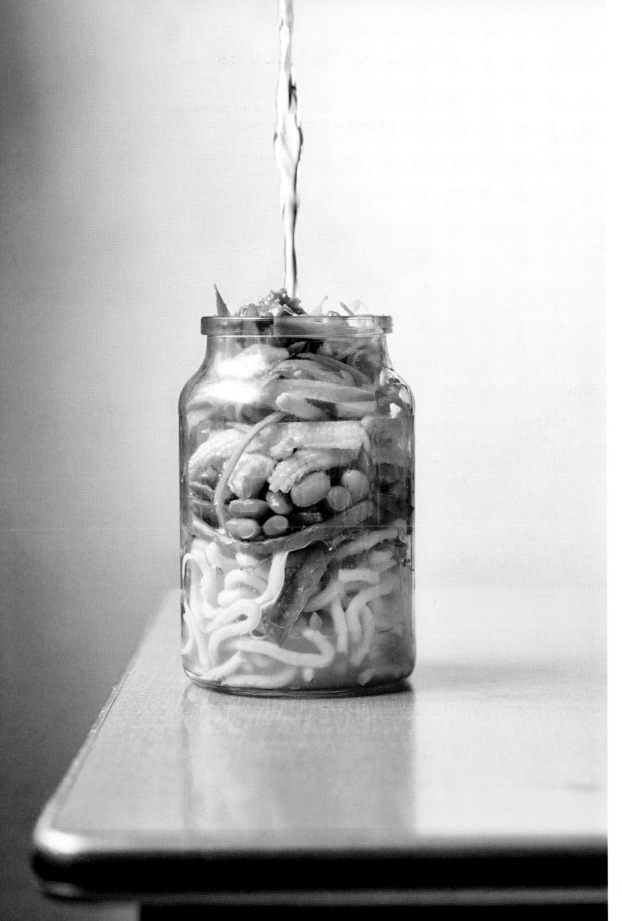

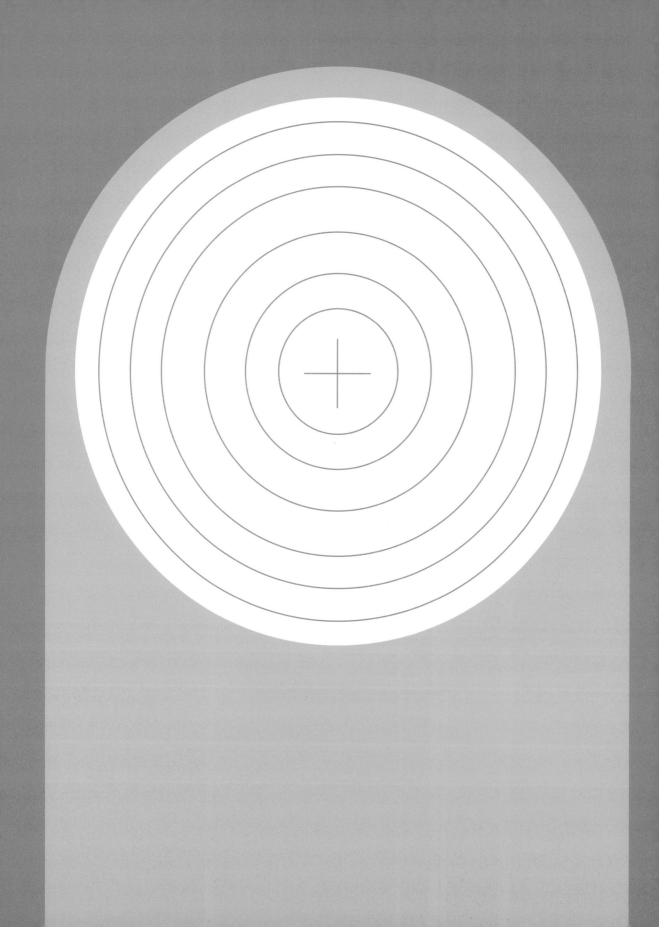

SNACKS

Feeding* your cravings, the right way

There are some patients you meet and do not forget; Laura was one of these patients, a 36-year-old mother of three who found herself in a pre-diabetic state, desperate to shift the extra pounds. She was struggling to find the time and motivation to exercise and the weight gain had significantly affected her mood and self-esteem.

When we spoke in detail about what she ate for her main meals, I was pleasantly surprised; a range of gut-healthy plant-based foods such as fruit and vegetables, whole grains, legumes and pulses were the mainstay of her family's diet. But it was in moments of peace and quiet, away from her children, that she would delve into snack drawer at home. Crisps, chocolate bars, biscuits and fizzy drinks were therapy, allowing her to unwind and relax.

As a mother to young children, I understood her sentiments and motivations completely. At times snacks are a survival mechanism. I've lost track of the number of times I have found myself in the kitchen foraging for something ultra-processed: either, crispy, crunchy and salty or gooey, soft and sweet. But it's when our snack-dependent survival methods threaten our long-term gut health, and broader metabolic health (as was the case with Laura), that things really need to change.

I would like you to use this chapter firstly as a strategic opportunity for you to assess your own personal relationship with snacking. Is this relationship truly beneficial or detrimental to your long-term health? Is there room for improvement? Secondly, this chapter is an opportunity to inspire you to make your own gut-healthy snack items. From crispy chickpeas to baked kale crisps, these recipes will excite the senses and the taste buds. Importantly, the recipes in this chapter share some of the same textures as those ultra-processed sweet and salty snacks that hit the pleasure centres of our brains. However, unlike ultra-processed snacks, the snacks in this chapter are joyously fibre-dense, and therefore hopefully have the added bonus of enhancing your gut's microbial diversity.

In these recipes, I have been mindful of keeping the salt used to a minimum. I acknowledge wholeheartedly that salt adds flavour to food in a way that almost nothing else can. But excess salt has detrimental effects, like increased blood pressure, risk of heart attacks and strokes. The UK government suggests we eat no more than 6g a day, which is about a level teaspoon. The average Brit consumes about 8g a day.

Researchers at the organisation 'Action on Salt' point out that snacks which are specifically marketed as 'healthy' may in fact be sabotaging our long-term health due to the huge amounts of salt that they contain. Based on government guidelines, over half of the 'healthy' snacks on the market are considered high or extremely high in fat, salt and/or sugar. Some 'healthy' crisps were even found to be, by weight, saltier than seawater! Astounding.

The worst culprits in terms of salt content were snacks like lentil curls, chickpea puffs and corn nuts. Notice a pattern? If the product sounds like it should be healthy, people usually just assume it is. From my perspective, the best way that you can be sure that what you're eating is healthy is to cook your own gut-friendly snack items at home. This way, you control exactly what is goes into the snack, and therefore what goes into your body. Substituting crisps and biscuits for carrot sticks and hummus, apples and peanut butter, a handful of nuts or dried mango may seem difficult at first, but with persistence and time, you will notice the positive metabolic impact that a gut health-focused method of snacking has on your body.

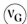

Tropical Sun Roast Chickpeas

SERVES 4

Plant Diversity
Score: 1.25

These are perfect for when you crave something salty. More fibre-dense than crisps, with a crunchy, firm texture which hits our brain's pleasure centre, this is a guilt-free hunger-buster snack. All-purpose seasoning is a busy cook's secret weapon and already has salt in, so there's no need to add extra. If you don't have any to hand you can use any spice blend of your choice: Chinese five-spice, curry powder, ras el hanout or za'atar all work well here.

—

1 x 400g (14oz) tin chickpeas, drained

1 tbsp vegetable oil

½ tsp all-purpose seasoning

½ tsp smoked paprika

1. Preheat the oven to 180°C fan/200°C/gas mark 6 and line a baking tray with a sheet of baking paper.

2. Lay the chickpeas on a large sheet of kitchen paper and rub the surface with another sheet. The idea is to dry the chickpeas completely and release the outer husk from some of them. The more of these husks you can discard, the crispier your final roasted chickpeas will be. Mix the chickpeas with the vegetable oil, all-purpose seasoning and paprika, then scatter the chickpeas over the paper-lined baking tray. Roast for 25–30 minutes, shaking the tray every 5 minutes or so to ensure the heat is distributed evenly and the chickpeas all brown uniformly. Allow to cool before serving.

Naga Nuts

SERVES 6–8

Plant Diversity
Score: 2

I keep these spicy, sweet nuts in my car to stave off those in-between-meals hunger pangs. Mr Naga hot pepper pickle is a wonderful (and extremely hot) chilli paste that pairs perfectly with the sweet, malty flavour of powdered jaggery. If you can't get powdered jaggery in your local supermarket; soft light brown sugar works well too. You can use any really hot chilli sauce you have to hand, or even red chilli powder.

—

350g (12oz/3 cups) unroasted cashews

1 tsp Mr Naga hot pepper pickle

2 tbsp powdered jaggery (or soft light brown sugar)

1 tsp vegetable oil

Salt, to taste

1. Preheat the oven to 160°C fan/180°C/gas mark 4 and line a large baking sheet with foil. Combine all the ingredients in a large mixing bowl and stir well to ensure that everything is coated evenly. Season with salt to taste. Toss the coated nuts on to the lined baking tray and spread them out evenly.

2. Roast for 20 minutes, stirring every 4–5 minutes to distribute the heat evenly. Remove from the oven and empty them out on to a sheet of baking paper placed on a wire rack. The more space they have to cool, the crispier they will be. Stir occasionally with a wooden spoon as they are cooling to allow any steam to escape. Store in jam jars. They will keep well for up to a fortnight.

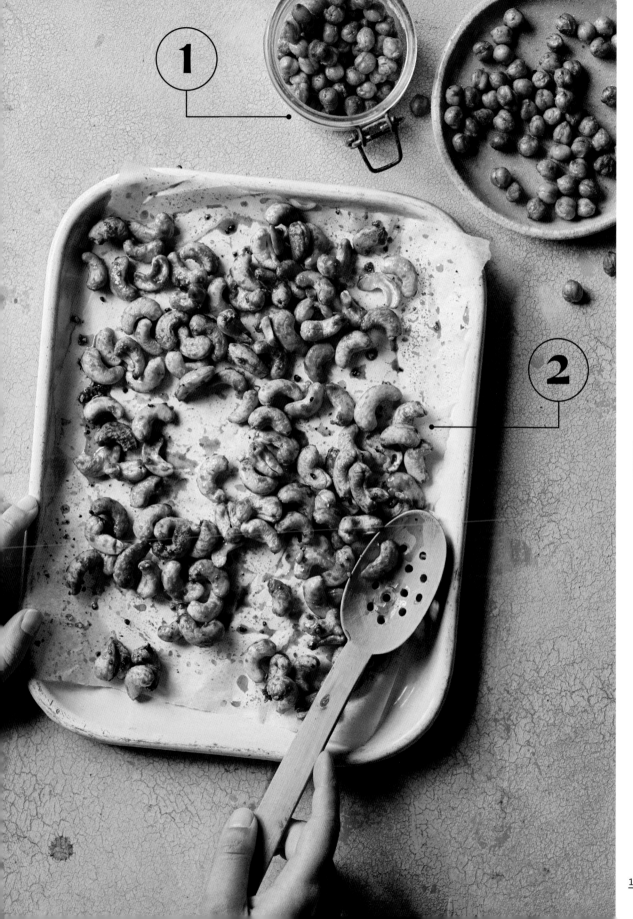

Coconut + Peanut Bars

MAKES 25

Plant Diversity
Score: 2

325g (11oz) desiccated coconut

100ml (3½fl oz/scant ½ cup) milk (or use your preferred plant-based milk)

1 x 400g (14oz) tin condensed milk

150g (5oz) dry roasted peanuts

150g (5oz) peanut butter

Imagine if the centre of a Bounty met a Reese's Peanut Butter Cup; you'd end up with a sort of coconut and peanut butter sandwich, but one where you only need a few bites to fill you up. Some sugar is used in the form of condensed milk here, but because it's so rich and filling you won't need more than one portion. The recipe makes a huge 25 portions for you to keep in the fridge, or if you're feeling particularly generous, to share with friends.

—

1. Start by putting the desiccated coconut into a saucepan and placing over a medium heat. When the coconut is warm and just starting to colour, add the milk and condensed milk. Stir everything well to combine and cook it for 5–7 minutes over a medium heat, stirring often. You know the mixture is ready when it looks sticky and moves away from the edge of the pan itself. Allow to cool completely. It will firm up a little as it cools.

2. Line a 20cm (8in) square brownie tin with baking paper. Take half the coconut mixture and press it down into the base of the tin. Now scatter over the dry roasted peanuts as evenly as possible, then spread over the peanut butter, spreading it all the way to the edges of the tin. Clean your hands and then layer with the remaining coconut mixture, pressing it down gently with either your clean hands or the back of a clean spoon that has been dipped in boiling water.

3. Allow to rest in the fridge for a couple of hours before cutting into 4cm (1½in) squares with a sharp knife. This will keep well in the fridge for 3–4 days.

the kitchen prescription

Peanut butter (The world's most popular spread)

+ Peanut butter is high in fat and calories – just 1 tablespoon contains about 120 calories. However, counting calories is a crude tool. While calorific, peanut butter is rich in unsaturated fats like oleic acid, and is a good source of magnesium, iron, copper, zinc and vitamins E and B.

+ Peanut butter is around 25 per cent protein, making

it an excellent plant-based source of protein.

+ Peanut butter is rich in antioxidants like p-coumarin and resveratrol, which show some health benefits in animals, though are yet to be studied in humans.

+ Buy varieties that are as close to 100 per cent peanut as possible as many brands add extra salt, palm oil and sugar.

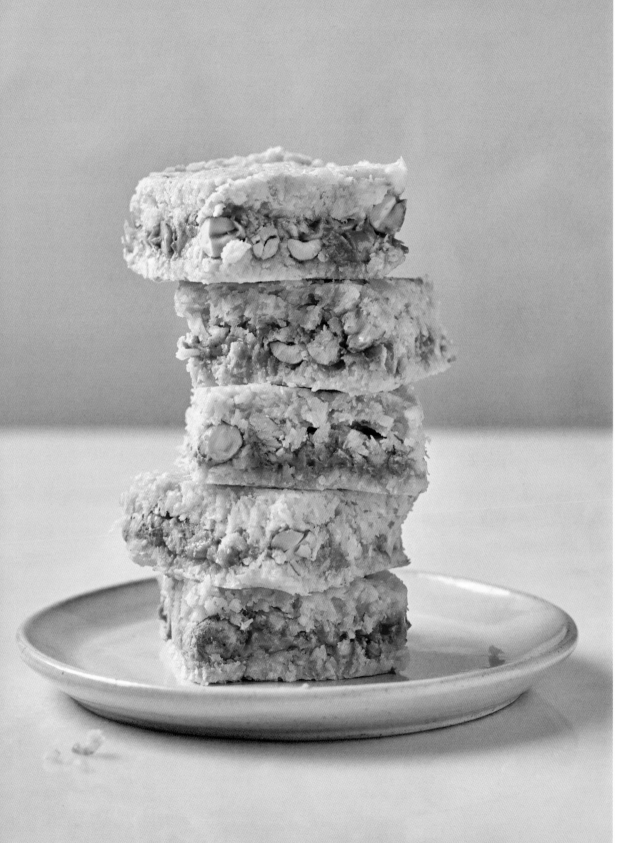

Panch Phoran Crackers with Cheese

Plant Diversity
Score: 3
Bonus Score: 2

These fibre-dense spiced crackers are the perfect accompaniment to probiotic cheese. Panch phoran, meaning 'five spices' in Bengali, is a combination of cumin, brown mustard, fenugreek, nigella and fennel seeds. To coax out these intense flavours I would recommend toasting the blend before roughly grinding it in a pestle and mortar.

—

100g (3½oz) wholewheat flour

100g (3½oz) plain white flour, plus extra for dusting

1 tbsp toasted panch phoran spices, roughly ground in a pestle and mortar

2 tbsp mixed seeds

4 tbsp olive oil, plus a little more for brushing

½ tsp sugar

1 tbsp black sesame seeds

Salt, to taste

Probiotic cheese of your choice (see below), to serve

BONUS GUT-FRIENDLY ADDITIONS

Thinly sliced Conference pear

Toasted walnuts

1. Preheat the oven to 180°C fan/200°C/gas mark 6 and line 2 large baking trays with baking paper. Combine both flours, the panch phoran spices, mixed seeds, oil and sugar in a large bowl. Season with salt and then slowly add about 100ml (3½fl oz/scant ½ cup) of water to form a firm dough: there is no need to knead the dough. You may need a little more or less water depending on the moisture content of the flour.

2. Roll the dough out on a lightly floured surface with a rolling pin. You are aiming for thin crackers, no more that 2mm (1⁄16in) thick. At this point you can either transfer the rolled dough on to the lined baking trays and bake it as 2 whole crackers, breaking into shards once cooked, or alternatively you can cut the dough into shapes of your choice, e.g. with a 8cm (3in) round or square cutter to make about 30 biscuits.

3. Before transferring to the oven, brush the surface of the cracker(s) with some more olive oil, then prick lightly with a fork and sprinkle over the sesame seeds. Bake for 15 minutes until crisp. Cool on a wire rack to ensure they are as crisp as possible. Serve with a selection of probiotic cheeses and pear and walnuts if you like.

the kitchen prescription

Cheese

+ Fermented milk products have been produced in various regions across the globe as far back as 10,000 BC.

+ Not all cheese you buy has probiotic content. Cheeses that have been aged and then heated, such as some supermarket brands of Cheddar, lose their probiotic superpowers.

+ Fermented cheeses with probiotic potential include both soft and hard cheese varieties. Labneh, cottage cheese, Swiss cheese, edam, provolone, Gouda, caciocavallo, aged traditional Cheddars, Parmigiano Reggiano, Pecorino Romano, Emmental, stinky blue cheese – take your pick.

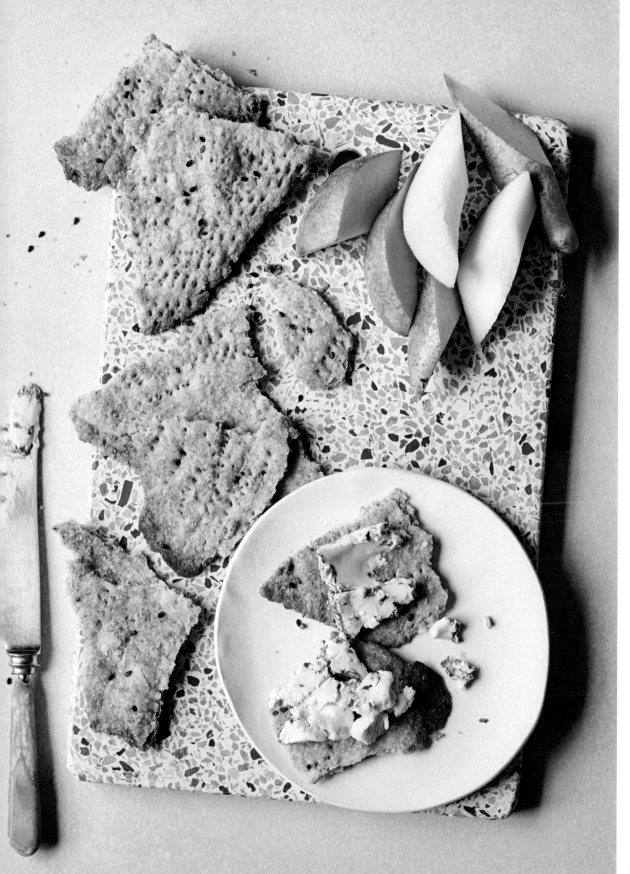

Kale Sesame Seaweed Crisps

SERVES 2-4

Plant Diversity
Score: 3

The definition of umami, these seaweed crisps are savoury, moreish and incredibly addictive. This recipe is worth a try for any readers who find themselves continually reaching for a packet of cheese and onion crisps. If you cannot get hold of dulse, try snipping up sheets of nori instead.

—

175g (6oz) kale

1 tsp sesame oil

1 tsp vegetable oil

1 tsp dried dulse seaweed or 1 roughly chopped sheet of nori seaweed

1 tsp sesame seeds

Flaky sea salt (not too much)

1. Preheat the oven to 130°C fan/150°C/gas mark 2. Line a large baking tray with baking paper or foil.

2. Cut out the thick stalks from the kale, leaving just the leaves. In a large bowl, toss together the kale leaves, sesame oil, vegetable oil, seaweed and sesame seeds and season with salt to taste. Ensure everything is combined well before transferring to the prepared baking tray and spreading as evenly as possible. Bake in the oven for 25–30 minutes, stirring every 8 minutes or so to ensure that the kale all browns and crisps up evenly.

---
the kitchen prescription

Seaweed

+ In Japan, about one fifth of meals contain seaweed. Edible seaweed can be classified into three groups: Chlorophyta (green), Phaeophyceae (brown) and Rhodophyta (red) algae.

+ Dulse (Palmaria palmata) is a nutrient-dense red seaweed with a mineral, oceanic taste. When cooked, some think it tastes smoky, like bacon. You can try it sprinkled over salad, fried eggs and popcorn, in mayonnaise dressings, melted into butter, served with fish...there are literally hundreds of uses.

+ Seaweed contains active polysaccharide fibres like alginate and fucoidan (thought to have cancer-reducing qualities), polyphenols like phlorotannins (thought to possess antioxidant, anti-inflammatory, anticancer and antidiabetic properties) and carotenoids like fucoxanthin (a potent antioxidant). These active compounds may also possess antimicrobial, blood pressure-lowering and bone protective properties.

+ Don't overdo it, though, as seaweed also has a fair bit of iodine in it, which in large quantities can have a negative impact on health.

110

Chilli Belly Popcorn

SERVES 4

Plant Diversity
Score: 2

Many varieties of shop-bought popcorn, cooked in a vat of oil and then covered in sugar and salt, are, unfortunately, not going to be particularly good for you. However, this home-made, freshly popped version is a different matter altogether. Popcorn is a whole grain; the maize kernel makes popcorn really high in dietary fibre, and therefore an excellent snack item. Just don't hide the health benefits by adding too much salt and sugar to your popcorn. I get around this by using spices and herbs to my advantage, but experiment with different options until you find your signature combination. Curry powder, all-purpose seasoning, Parmesan cheese, cayenne pepper or even nutritional yeast are all lovely additions to the popped whole grain.

—

2 tbsp sunflower oil

100g (3½oz/½ cup) popcorn kernels

50g (2oz) melted butter

1 tsp paprika

½ tsp chilli powder

1 tsp garlic granules

1 sprig of rosemary, leaves finely chopped

Salt, to taste

1. Find a large saucepan with a well-fitting lid and pour in the oil. Place the pan over a medium heat; when the oil is hot, add the popcorn kernels and rapidly put the lid on. Swill the pan around to distribute the heat and the popcorn kernels will start popping. Over the next minute or two the popping will be rapid – gently shake the pan around by moving it back and forth over the hob to help distribute the heat evenly. Once the popping slows to several seconds between pops, remove the pan from the heat, remove the lid and empty the popcorn out immediately into a wide bowl. This will mean that all the kernels pop and nothing burns.

2. Melt the butter in a small saucepan; once it starts to foam, add the paprika, chilli powder, garlic granules, rosemary and salt to taste. Drizzle the melted spiced butter over the popcorn and toss well to distribute all over.

SNACKS

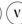 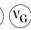

FRO-YO Fibre Bark

SERVES 6

Plant Diversity
Score: 5.25

Occasionally at snack time I love nothing more than to reach for the ice cream in the freezer. Here is my take on a gut-healthy ice cream (the king of treats), a fibre-dense dried mango and goji berry bark. It satisfies the ice-cream craving in me while simultaneously feeding the gut microbiome. You can try other toppings such as pineapple and passion fruit, or fresh berries and white chocolate chips, or even roughly chopped pistachio nuts and dark chocolate chips.

—

350g (12oz) strained full-fat live Greek yoghurt (or plant-based yoghurt)

1 tbsp maple syrup

1 tsp rosewater (optional)

¼ tsp ground cardamom (optional)

30g (1oz) dried goji berries

50g (2oz) dried mango, roughly chopped

15g (½oz) slivered pistachios or other nuts

10g (¼oz) toasted coconut shavings

15g (½oz) dried cranberries

1. Combine the Greek yoghurt, maple syrup, rosewater and ground cardamom (if using) in a large bowl and stir well to combine.

2. Line a large flat dinner plate or baking tray with baking paper and pour the yoghurt mixture on top. Spread the yoghurt out on the plate. You can have it thinner or thicker according to your preference; I tend to go for about 1cm (½in) thick. Sprinkle the goji berries, mango, pistachios, coconut and cranberries artfully over the yoghurt. Cover the plate or tray loosely with foil and place in the freezer for at least 12 hours to firm up completely.

3. When you are ready to serve, break the frozen yoghurt into shards. Consume within about 10 minutes or it will start to melt.

the kitchen prescription

Goji berries, Wolfberries (Lycium barbarum)

+ Goji berries are very popular in the health food market. Considered by some to be the original superfood, they have been used for centuries in Chinese medicine.

+ Goji berries are abundant in biologically active compounds: polysaccharides, carotenoids like zeaxanthin (which give them their vivid colour) and phenolic acids like caffeic acid, which have antioxidant properties.

+ Small studies show that goji berries can have protective effects on our vision, stimulate the immune system, and protect the heart and nerves, although the studies are currently too small-scale to draw any concrete conclusions.

+ Although undoubtedly full of good stuff, the jury is still out on how much these little berries impact our health.

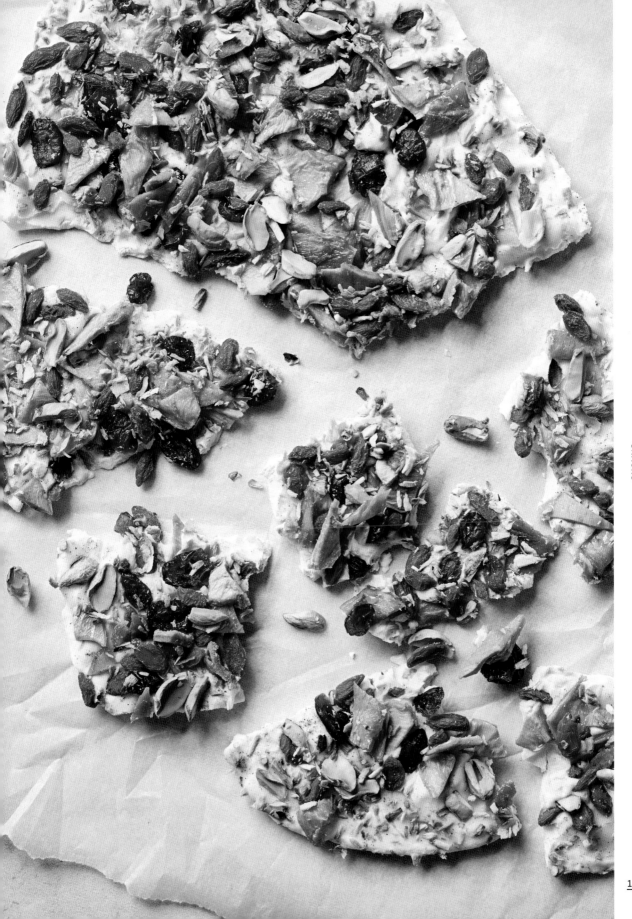

Toasted Pine Nut + Ginger Oaty Cookies

MAKES 12

Plant Diversity
Score: 2

Author and expert baker Alice Medrich puts it perfectly when she says, 'there's a cookie for every mood and motivation, personality and predilection'. She's right. These oaty, nutty cookies will gain a special place in your heart, and by virtue of their fibre content, your gut too. Naturally, they are still a cookie, so look at these as a treat item, not to be eaten in excess.

—

60g (2½oz/⅔ cup) porridge oats

60g (2½oz/½ cup) plain flour

1 tsp baking powder

1 egg, beaten

75g (2¾oz) powdered jaggery (or soft light brown sugar)

50g (2oz) melted coconut oil or butter

50g (2oz) toasted pine nuts

50g (2oz) crystallised ginger, finely diced

1. Preheat the oven to 180°C fan/200°C/gas mark 6. Line a large baking tray with baking paper.

2. Combine the porridge oats, plain flour and baking powder in a bowl and stir well: this is the dry mix. In a separate bowl, beat together the egg, jaggery and coconut oil until well combined. Pour this mixture over the dry mix and combine well with a wooden spoon. Refrigerate the mixture for 1 hour.

3. Divide the cookie dough into 12 equal-sized portions. Shape them with your hands into walnut-shaped balls and then press them gently to flatten. Place the cookies on the lined tray and gently stud the surface with the pine nuts and ginger pieces.

4. Transfer to the oven and bake for about 12 minutes, or until they are golden and crisp at the edges. They will spread as they cook, so leave some space between them and if your baking tray is not big enough, use two instead of one. Remove from the oven and allow to cool slightly before eating. They will keep for a week stored in an airtight container.

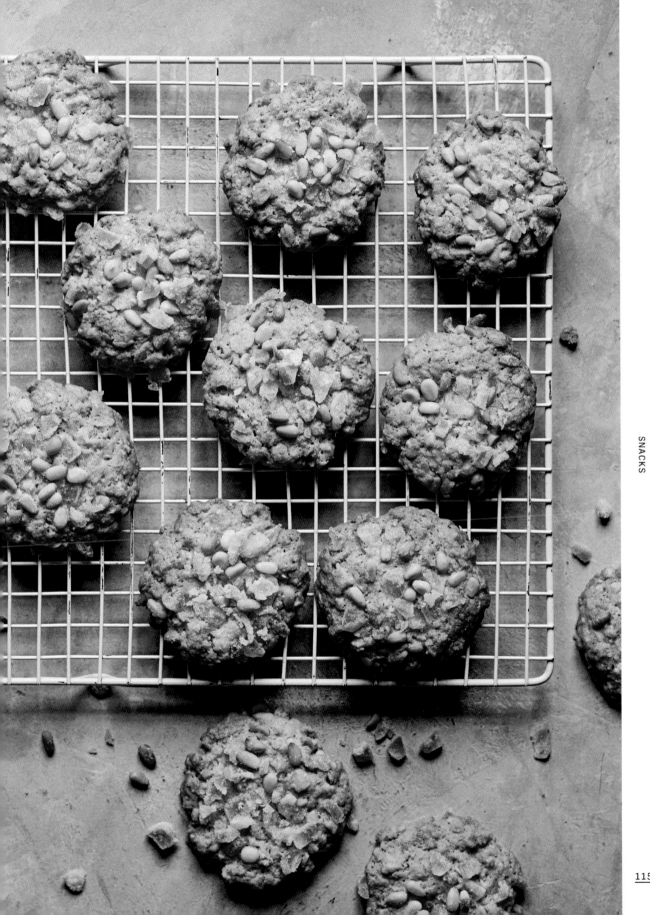

Snack Attack Boiled Eggs

MAKES 2

I love boiled eggs. There's a process that I like to follow when I eat them: the ritual of cracking the shell, cutting the egg in half, and scattering seasoning over the white and yolk calms me while the egg itself fills up my belly until the next meal. These recipes are designed for two boiled eggs and work well with either soft-centred or hard-boiled eggs, whichever you prefer. Inspired by flavours from around the globe, these recipes are not only filling, but also far better for you than reaching for a pack of crisps or a chocolate bar.

Topping 1: Asian Seeded

1 tsp toasted pumpkin seeds
1 tsp black sesame seeds
1 tsp toasted sunflower seeds
½ tsp Chinese five-spice
Pinch of salt (optional)

Mix all the ingredients together and scatter over halved eggs.

Topping 2: Spicy Soy

2 tsp dark soy sauce
2 tsp chilli oil (I like Lao Gan Ma crispy chillies in oil)
1 tsp finely chopped toasted peanuts
3 chives, finely chopped

Halve the eggs. Drizzle over the soy sauce, followed by the chilli oil. Top with the toasted peanuts and chives.

Topping 3: Cheese + Herbs

1 tbsp cream cheese, labneh or thick Greek yoghurt
2 tsp finely chopped parsley (or other herbs of your choice)
½ tsp za'atar (or a pinch of dried oregano)
Zest of ½ lemon
Pinch of salt (optional)
Drizzle of extra-virgin olive oil, to finish

Mix the labneh with the parsley and spoon over the halved eggs. Sprinkle over the za'atar and lemon zest. Season with salt to taste, drizzle over some olive oil and enjoy.

Topping 4: Coronation-style

½ tsp curry powder
1 tbsp crème fraîche
Few grinds of black pepper
Pinch of salt (optional)
2 tsp mango chutney
1 tsp finely chopped coriander

Combine the curry powder with the crème fraîche, black pepper and salt to taste. Spoon the mixture over the halved eggs, then top with the mango chutney and chopped coriander.

the kitchen prescription

Eggs

+ There is no real recommended limit to how many eggs people should eat; an array of studies show conflicting results about how, or even whether, eggs affect the health of our heart.

+ What we do know is that eggs are a good source of protein, energy and vitamins D and B. The concerns centre around the fact that the yolks of eggs are rich in cholesterol. But the cholesterol in eggs is not thought to have a significant effect on blood cholesterol. To lower blood cholesterol, it is much more important to limit the amount of saturated fat in the diet.

+ Overall, I would recommend a moderate-to-low intake of eggs (approx 1–2 per week). They are delicious and I don't avoid them, but there are also plenty of other sources of protein that you can opt for, for instance from plants or nuts.

After School Gut Love

Rather than a recipe, this is a little log of some of the gut-healthy snacks I feed my famished children when they come home from school. They are 'pick and mix' type snack ideas for children, as well adults coming home from a hard day of work. I have written them to serve as some inspiration for you...a way of avoiding those dreaded packets of crisps and cookies in moments of starvation.

—

Monday
+ ½ green apple, thinly sliced, and 1 tbsp peanut butter
+ 2–3 dates
+ Handful of cashews (unsalted)
+ 3 tbsp pomegranate seeds

Tuesday
+ 2 sesame-coated breadsticks
+ 6 carrot sticks and 1 tbsp hummus
+ 2 squares of dark chocolate
+ Approximately 4 strawberries

Wednesday
+ Small bunch of grapes
+ 6–8 almonds
+ 1 tangerine
+ 1 live strawberry yoghurt

Thursday
+ 3 dried figs
+ 8 raspberries
+ 50g (2oz) mature Cheddar cheese
+ 1 tbsp toasted pumpkin seeds

Friday
+ 4 dried apricots
+ ½ x 400g (14oz) tin pineapple or peach slices (in juice, not syrup)
+ ½ cucumber, sliced into batons
+ Handful of walnuts

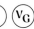

Gut Boost Energy Bars

MAKES 16

Plant Diversity
Score: 6

Dates, carrots, almond butter and tahini are the foundation of these nutritious energy bars. All their sweetness comes from the natural sugars in the dates, rather than any added sweetness from refined sugar. Feel free to adapt and add any nuts, dried fruit or mixed seeds – whatever you fancy. Chocolate lovers can dust the surface with cocoa powder too. Once they are ready, keep them in the fridge to grab and go.

—

3 carrots, grated

15 pitted Medjool dates, soaked in boiling water for 15 minutes

100g (3½oz/1 cup) toasted jumbo oats (or gluten-free toasted jumbo oats)

1 tbsp milled flaxseeds

1 tbsp toasted sesame seeds, plus extra for sprinkling

125g (4oz) almond butter

2 tbsp tahini

1 tbsp apricot jam, to glaze

1. Put the carrots into a small saucepan and place over a medium heat. Cook the carrots for 3–4 minutes so the moisture steams away and they lose their rawness, then allow to cool.

2. Drain the dates thoroughly of any excess water, then chop them roughly and add to a bowl with the carrots. Now add the oats, flaxseeds, sesame seeds, almond butter and tahini. Stir everything really well to combine. The mixture should be reasonably firm; if it is not, just add a little extra oats.

3. Press the mixture into a 25cm (10in) square cake tin lined with baking paper. Brush the surface with apricot jam and add an extra sprinkling of sesame seeds to give a sheen. Refrigerate for a few hours before cutting into squares or bar shapes as you like. They will keep for a week stored in an airtight container.

the kitchen prescription

Dates (Phoenix dactylifera)

+ Medjool dates are known as 'the fruit of kings'. This title is not surprising given their health benefits.

+ Dates are rich in polyphenols, carotenoids and lignans, compounds that possess antioxidant properties and help manage the risk of developing a plethora of chronic diseases.

+ Dates are also packed full of micronutrients like phosphorus, potassium, calcium, magnesium and vitamin K – they are pretty fibre-dense too.

+ Dates are an excellent replacement for refined sugar. If you blend dates with water you can make a syrup with a lower fructose content than many other sweeteners.

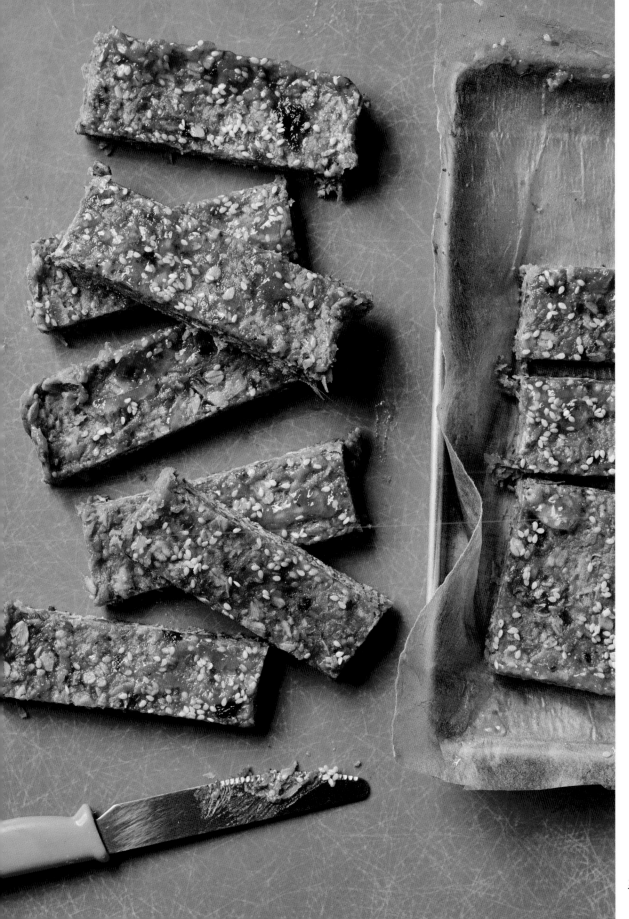

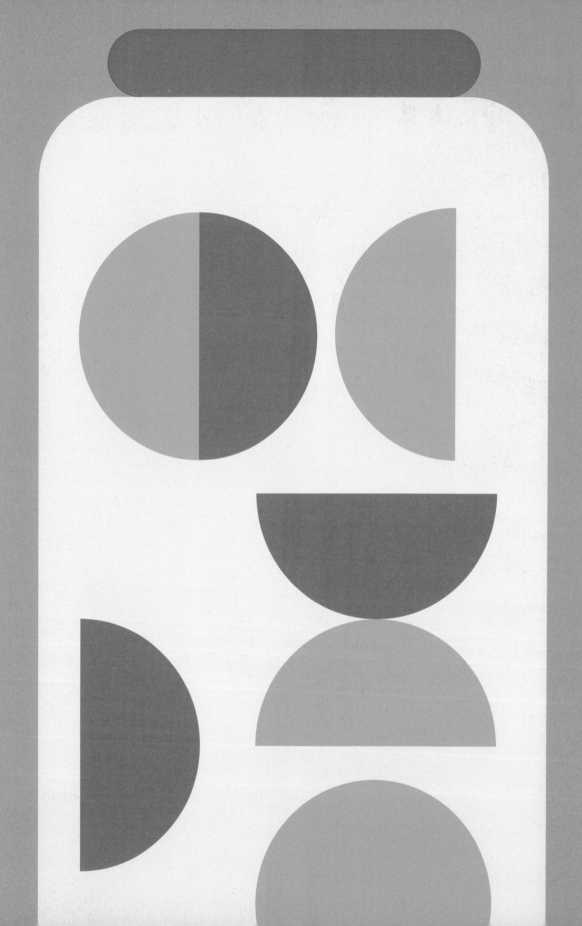

FREEZER

CUPBOARD

STORE +

The hidden secret to good gut health

A person's freezer shelves and cupboards are a sort of culinary fingerprint; an identifiable and unique curation of ingredients. However, they are often considered the backstage areas of our kitchen. We treat our fridges like the stars of the show when trying to figure out what to make for dinner, but forget that the ingredients housed in the freezer and storecupboard can form the foundations to achieving good gut health. Through the recipes in this chapter, I will demonstrate that by using just storecupboard and freezer items, you can make some incredible, gut-friendly meals and dishes. From vibrant soups to aromatic lentil dishes – even salads can be made from the stuff in these two underappreciated kitchen zones.

To maximise the gut-friendly contents of your storecupboard, here are my tips on how to keep it stocked.

+ **Dried and tinned lentils/beans:** green lentils, brown lentils, red lentils, chana dal (split chickpeas) and beluga lentils are all good in their dried form. Add tins of Puy, green and brown lentils, chickpeas (white and brown varieties), kidney beans, black-eyed peas, pinto beans and fava beans.

+ **Dried grains and rice:** bulgur wheat, quinoa, spelt, freekeh, pearl barley, brown rice and wild rice (dried or cooked in packets) can provide the carbohydrate foundation for so many dishes. For more on the beneficial types of dietary carbohydrates see page 15.

- **Various forms of pasta and dried noodles:** like rice and pulses, these are the foundational ingredients upon which you can build your Italian pasta dishes and Asian noodle delights. Try fibre-rich varieties like wholewheat pasta or soba noodles where possible.

- **Tinned fruit:** mango slices, grapefruit segments, pineapple slices and tinned peaches (buy them 'in juice', not syrup). In moderation, these are great for kids to snack on, and provide long-lasting access to nutrients found in fruits that are more expensive when bought fresh. For more on how to use these see the desserts chapter (pages 228–47).

- **Tinned fish:** anchovies (an umami staple), tinned sardines and mackerel (an incredibly cheap option) and tins of tuna (in spring water rather than oil).

- **Other essential storecupboard items:** coconut milk, tinned cherry tomatoes, stock cubes, etc. are essential basics worth stocking up on.

Rather than filling the freezer with frozen pizzas, ready meals or burger patties I try to opt for frozen 'whole' foods. Here is how I organise my freezer.

- **Frozen vegetables (less exotic):** peas, carrots, spinach, broccoli, frozen chopped onions, sweetcorn cobs, mixed root vegetables such as celeriac, swede and squash.

- **Frozen vegetables (more exotic):** frozen kale, edamame beans, okra, fenugreek leaves, molokhia leaves, shredded fresh frozen coconut. If you've ever glanced at the price of these vegetables when fresh you'll understand why I prefer frozen for my more exotic recipe requirements.

- **Frozen fruit:** strawberries, bananas, orange segments, cranberries (at Christmas), sometimes mango and papaya chunks. Perfect for yoghurt toppings, home-made ice cream etc.

- **Other miscellaneous frozen essentials:** garlic and ginger in cubes, filo pastry, puff pastry, a jointed chicken. These frozen items are highly convenient when cooking for a family.

- **Pre-cooked meals:** soups, frozen home-made lasagne and curries. Batch-cook and then freeze in portions to make your own home-made frozen ready meals.

This is just a rough guide, and I urge you to personalise your storecupboard and freezer to your own taste and preferences. My hope is that after trying out some of these recipes, you will no longer consider the storecupboard and freezer places where food in your kitchen goes to live out its retirement years, and more of an active part of your gut-friendly culinary practice. The recipes in this chapter are wonderfully resourceful, and by cooking them often and adapting them to your tastes, you will automatically start populating your storecupboard and freezer in a more effective way.

Once you start using your storecupboard and freezer to their maximum potential, there's no going back; it's not only good for your gut but also for your wallet, as many of the items are significantly cheaper than fresh produce. So, spare a thought for the gut-healthy tins of protein-rich beans or the ancient but still perfectly useful dried lentils lurking in the cupboard, or indeed the vitamin-rich pack of frozen green beans gathering ice at the back of the freezer, just there, under the ice lollies and fish fingers.

South Indian-style Chickpea + Mango Salad

SERVES 4

Plant Diversity
Score: 5.25

1 x 400g (14oz) tin white chickpeas

1 x 400g (14oz) tin black chickpeas (kala chana)

2 tbsp olive oil

8 curry leaves (ideally fresh, but use dried if you can't get them fresh)

Thumb-sized piece of ginger, peeled and grated

1 tsp mustard seeds

1–2 green chillies, finely chopped

½ tsp cumin seeds

½ tsp asafoetida (optional)

75g (2¾oz) grated coconut or 2 tbsp desiccated coconut

250g (9oz) finely diced fresh or tinned mango

Juice of 1 lime

Salt, to taste

In many ways, this dish sums up the way I eat: an explosion of flavour at minimal cost and totally gut-loving. I use three tins here: white chickpeas, black chickpeas and tinned mango. The grated coconut can be bought frozen from Asian food stores, or you can use desiccated coconut from your storecupboard.

—

1. Start by draining the black and white chickpeas from the tins and running them under warm water to refresh them.

2. Heat the olive oil in a pan over a medium heat. When the oil is hot but not smoking, add the curry leaves and ginger, followed by the mustard seeds, green chillies, cumin seeds and asafoetida (if using). Stir well to combine.

3. When the mustard seeds start popping, add the chickpeas and season with salt to taste. Allow the chickpeas to warm through for a few minutes before taking the pan off the heat. Cool slightly before adding the coconut, mango and lime juice. Serve warm, at room temperature or cold.

---

the kitchen prescription

Chickpeas (Cicer arietinum L.)

+ Chickpeas are full of plant-based protein and gut-healthy fibre.

+ Black chickpeas in particular are packed with gut-friendly raffinose, a type of fibre that is fermented in the colon by a beneficial bacteria called Bifidobacterium. As bacteria break down raffinose, a short-chain fatty acid called butyrate is produced, which exerts many beneficial effects on the wall of the colon.

+ Both tinned and dried chickpeas (black and white) contain resistant starch, which is released slowly into the bloodstream, so you won't experience such sudden surges in blood sugar.

+ Chickpeas are full of a plant sterol called sitosterol, which is similar to cholesterol. It acts by interfering with the body's absorption of cholesterol and therefore has a positive impact on blood cholesterol levels.

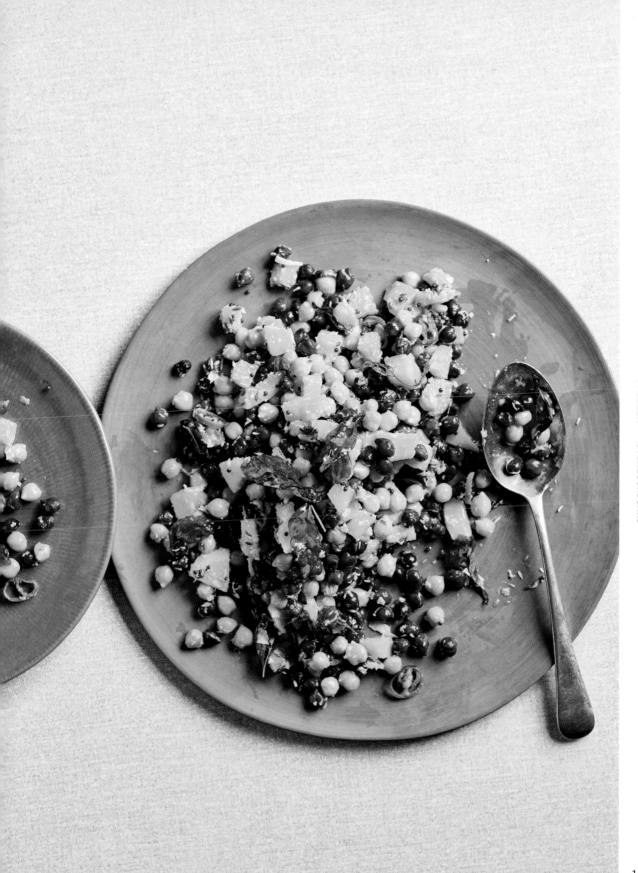

Tuna + White Beans with Miso Orange Dressing

SERVES 2

Plant Diversity
Score: 5
Bonus Score: 1

This dish is a reminder that with the addition of a few fresh ingredients, a tin of tuna and a tin of cannellini beans can be transformed into a dish that no one would ever realise is constructed from the inhabitants of the darkest depths of your pantry.

—

1 x 125g (4oz) tin tuna, drained

1 x 400g (14oz) tin cannellini beans, drained

Segments of 1 fresh large orange or 150g (5oz) tinned mandarin segments

Handful of finely chopped parsley

Handful of pitted black olives (from a jar)

FOR THE ONION

½ red onion, thinly sliced (can be frozen and defrosted)

Juice ½ lemon

½ tsp sugar

Pinch of salt

FOR THE DRESSING

½ tsp gluten-free miso paste

½ red chilli, finely chopped

1 tsp honey

1 tbsp olive oil

2 tbsp orange juice

BONUS GUT-FRIENDLY ADDITION

Generous handful of rocket, spinach or watercress leaves

1. Start by combining the onion with the lemon juice, sugar and salt: give everything a good scrunch in your hands to soften the onions and help release their pink colour.

2. Mix the miso paste with the chilli, honey, olive oil and orange juice in a small bowl. Whisk to form a dressing.

3. Combine the tuna, cannellini beans, orange segments, parsley and olives in a small bowl. Pour over the miso dressing and toss well to combine. Finish by scattering over the red onion slices. Serve immediately with a handful of leaves if you like.

the kitchen prescription

Tuna

+ There are no carbohydrates in tuna, just protein. Tuna is an excellent source of vitamin B (in particular niacin, which supports the nervous system) and omega-3 fatty acids.

+ Tinned tuna has about half the amount of vitamin D when compared with fresh tuna.

+ Tinned tuna can come in brine, oil or water – varieties in oil tends to be higher in fat while those packed in brine are high in salt. Try to buy tuna in spring water.

+ To buy sustainably sourced tinned tuna always look for the MSC label.

+ Tuna can be high in mercury content, so limit how much of it you eat. Light or skipjack tuna are lower in mercury than bigeye or albacore tuna.

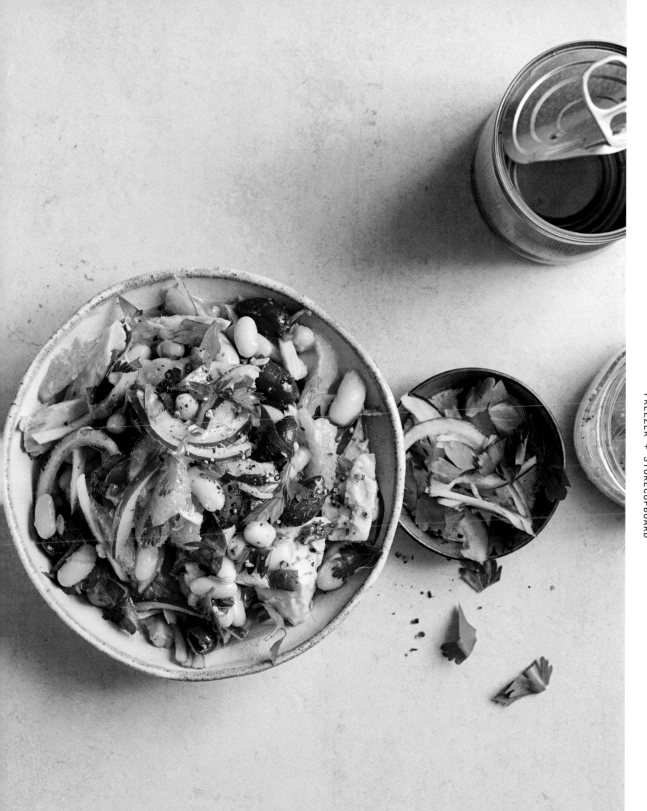

Grapefruit + Lentils with Thai-style Dressing

Plant Diversity
Score: 3.75
Bonus Score: 4 or more

1 x 400g (14oz) tin green lentils (235g/8oz drained weight)

1 x 540g (19oz) tin grapefruit segments (290g/10oz drained weight)

½ red onion, thinly sliced

2 garlic cloves

1 tbsp soft light brown sugar

2 tbsp fish sauce

3 tbsp lime juice

1–2 bird's-eye chillies, finely chopped

3 tbsp grapefruit juice (reserved from the tin)

Handful of fresh coriander leaves, roughly chopped

BONUS GUT-FRIENDLY ADDITIONS

Grated carrots, cucumbers sticks, sliced peppers, green beans, or even a handful of beansprouts

The tinned lentils and grapefruit in this recipe soak up the flavour of the umami-rich fish sauce like a sponge, mingling the bitterness of the grapefruit with a touch of sugar and fiery chilli heat.

—

1. Drain the lentils in a sieve, discarding the water from the tin. Run them though some warm water to refresh them. Drain the grapefruit, saving the juice. Place the lentils and grapefruit in a serving bowl along with the sliced onion.

2. Pound the garlic cloves in a pestle and mortar along with the sugar until smooth. Add the fish sauce, lime juice, chillies and reserved grapefruit juice from the tin and stir well to combine. Spoon the dressing over the grapefruit and tinned lentils, then scatter over the coriander leaves and serve. Add extra veg for increased plant diversity if you like.

the kitchen prescription

Grapefruit (Citrus x paradisi)

+ Grapefruit is a fantastic source of vitamin C, which is beneficial for the optimal functioning of our immune system.

+ It is rich in fibre, which means it makes us feel full for longer. There is also evidence to suggest that eating grapefruit regularly may help reduce insulin resistance and therefore reduce the risk of developing type 2 diabetes.

+ Grapefruit is heart-healthy, helping regulate cholesterol and blood pressure. Some studies show that grapefruit may reduce stroke risk, particularly in women, although more research is needed to work out the reasons behind this.

+ Grapefruit also contains several antioxidants, vitamin C, beta-carotene, lycopene and flavonoids, all of which work together to protect our body's cells from damage.

+ When buying tinned grapefruit, try to opt for the varieties in unsweetened grapefruit juice.

Pea, Coconut +
Lemongrass Soup

SERVES 1

Plant Diversity
Score: 2.75
Bonus Score: 3

There is a part of my brain that is completely dedicated to fantasies of sitting on a sun-kissed veranda, breaking open fresh peas in their pods while watching my children come and steal the sweet, freshly shelled jewels from their bowl. The reality is that I live in London and fresh peas in their shells are unlikely to be found in my kitchen. Happily, all that gut-friendly green pea glory has been harvested for me and sits reliably in my freezer, ready to be made into this delightful soup.

—

1 x 400ml (14fl oz) tin full-fat coconut milk

½ lemongrass stalk (15g/½oz), bruised lightly

200ml (7fl oz/generous ¾ cup) vegetable stock

1 red chilli, roughly chopped

Thumb-sized piece of ginger, peeled and roughly chopped

350g (12oz) frozen petit pois

2 tsp fish sauce

Zest and juice of 1 lime

Salt, to taste

BONUS GUT-FRIENDLY ADDITIONS

For an extra hit of plant-based diversity, steam 100g (3½oz) pak choi leaves, a handful of mangetout and green beans for 2 minutes.

Add the steamed vegetables to the pea broth just before serving.

1. Put the coconut milk, lemongrass, vegetable stock, red chilli and ginger in a saucepan and simmer gently for 15 minutes to allow the flavours to infuse the coconut milk.

2. Remove the lemongrass and ginger (and the chilli if you don't like it too hot) from the coconut milk and add the frozen petit pois. Bring back to a simmer and cook the petit pois for just 1–2 minutes, then remove from the heat.

3. Transfer the mixture to a blender and blitz to a smooth purée. Return the broth to the saucepan and season with fish sauce and salt to taste. Finish with the lime zest and juice. The broth is ready to be eaten; top with a few extra steamed green vegetables if you prefer.

FREEZER + STORE CUPBOARD

Charred Corn with Mango Chutney Butter

MAKES 8

Plant Diversity
Score: 2.5
Bonus Score: 1

4 whole (or 8 half) frozen corn on the cobs

50g (2oz) butter

1 heaped tbsp gluten-free mango chutney

1 red chilli, finely chopped

Zest and juice of 1 lime

1 tsp chaat masala (optional)

Green tips of 2 spring onions, thinly sliced into rounds

Handful of fresh coriander, finely chopped

Salt, to taste

Frozen corn on the cob is a staple in my kitchen. Both my seven-year-old and my baby love eating it with their dinner, which is why I always have some lurking around. In this recipe a little extra tender love and care transforms the humble frozen corn into a grown-up, gut-loving dish.

—

1. Cook the corn on the cob according to the packet instructions – this usually involves boiling for about 6–8 minutes from frozen. Drain the corn and allow it to steam dry for a few minutes.

2. Melt the butter in a saucepan and add the mango chutney, chilli and lime zest. Remove from the heat. Turn your gas cooker on to full flame and carefully grab a corn cob with some tongs. Hold the cob in the naked flame, rotating slightly to ensure that all sides of the sweetcorn are charred. (If you don't have a gas hob you can do this under a hot grill or in griddle pan.)

3. Brush the corn cobs with the mango chutney butter and sprinkle over the chaat masala (if using), sliced spring onion and coriander. Season with a little salt and spritz with lime juice before serving.

Corn (Zea mays L.)

+ Although it is usually considered a vegetable, corn is in fact a whole grain.

+ It is rich in dietary fibre and vitamins C and B, as well as plant sterols thought to have a positive effect on body cholesterol.

+ Lutein and zeaxanthin are two carotenoids found in corn. These compounds contribute to good eye health by protecting a part of the back of the eye called the macula.

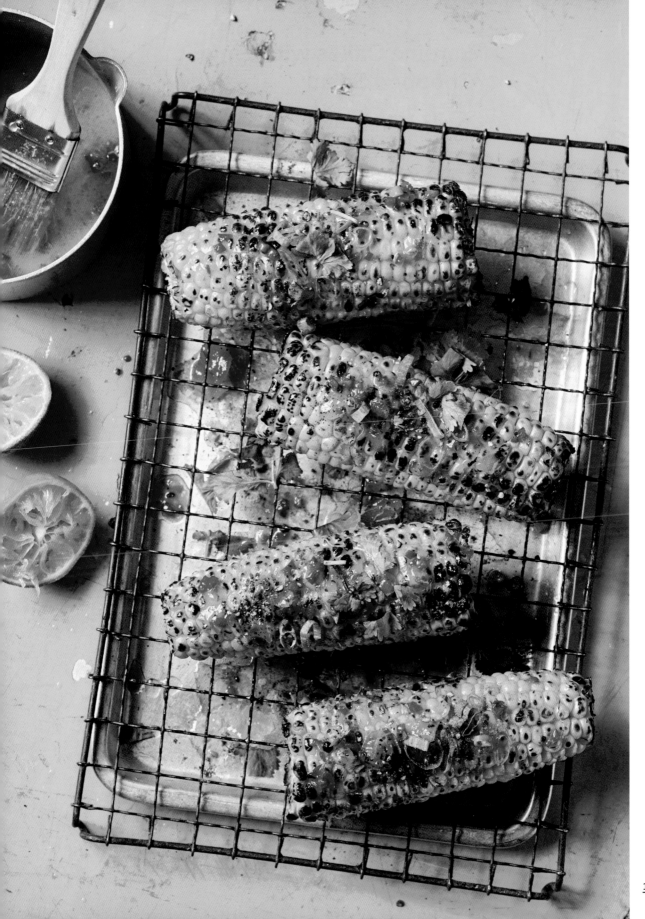

Sardine Cakes with Zingy Chopped Salad

MAKES 8 (SERVES 4)

Plant Diversity
Score: 5.75

These fishcakes showcase sardines in a way that will change the way you look at these versatile little storecupboard fish. They are completely addictive umami bombs; I guarantee that after you have had your first morsel of intense deliciousness, you'll be licking your fingers and eyeing up how many are left on the plate.

The irresistibility of this dish is courtesy of katta sambol paste, a popular Sri Lankan condiment made from shallots and chillies. I would suggest that you get your hands on a jar by searching online or heading to your local Asian supermarket. You can use plain red chilli paste or harissa paste as a suitable alternatives.

—

2 x 120g (4oz) tins sardines (in oil, not tomato sauce)

2 heaped tsp katta sambol paste (or 1 tsp red chilli paste, or 2 tsp harissa)

400g (14oz) mashed potato

2 spring onions, thinly sliced

Handful of finely chopped coriander

3 tbsp plain flour

4 tsp vegetable oil

FOR THE SALAD

1 large tomato, finely diced

1 cucumber, finely diced

½ red onion, finely diced

8 mint leaves, thinly sliced

½ tsp red chilli powder

Juice of ½ lemon

Salt, to taste

1. Drain the oil from the sardines and place them in a bowl. (If you like, remove the backbone with the tip of a sharp knife.) Add the katta sambol paste, mashed potato, spring onions and chopped coriander and mix well to form a fishcake mixture. Chill for 15–20 minutes in the fridge.

2. Put the flour into a shallow bowl. Heat a non-stick frying pan over a medium heat with 1 teaspoon of vegetable oil. Lightly oil your fingers with a little vegetable oil and shape the fishcake mixture into 8 patties, about 8cm (3in) wide and 2cm (¾in) thick.

3. One by one, place the patties in the flour and coat both sides with a thin dusting of flour. Gently place the fishcakes in the hot frying pan and fry for a few minutes on each side until deep golden in colour. Do this in batches of two or three for ease.

4. Combine all the ingredients for the salad together in a bowl and mix well. Serve alongside the fishcakes. These patties make an excellent filling in burgers.

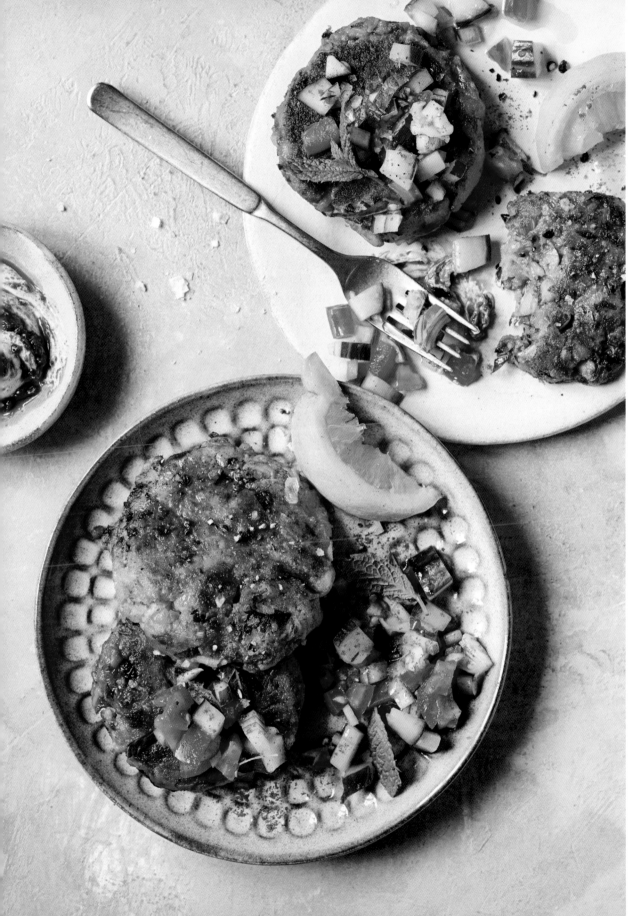

Curried Bean Swirl

SERVES 4-6

Plant Diversity
Score: 4.25

A recipe to showcase the versatility of both the storecupboard and the freezer – here filo pastry and fibre-dense tinned beans are celebrated in all their glory. It's a real showstopper, both in how it looks and tastes. Crack this recipe out when you're entertaining guests at short notice and don't want to spend a fortune on expensive ingredients, but still want to make their jaws hit the floor. You can use whichever tinned beans you have to hand.

—

2 x 400g (14oz) tins butter beans (or use chickpeas, red kidney beans or rosecoco beans)

1 tbsp olive oil

2 spring onions, finely chopped

2 tbsp your favourite jalfrezi/korma paste

100g (3½oz/1 cup) grated Cheddar cheese

8 sheets of filo pastry, defrosted

100g (3½oz) melted butter

2 tbsp mixed seeds

1. Preheat the oven to 170°C fan/190°C/gas mark 5 and line a baking sheet with baking paper. Drain the beans and refresh them in some warm water, then allow them to air dry for a little while.

2. Heat the olive oil in a frying pan over a medium heat and add the spring onions. When they start to turn golden, add the beans and curry paste. Allow the beans to cook through for a few minutes, before removing from the heat and leaving to cool. Add the grated cheese to the cooled beans and stir well. The filling for your pie is now ready.

3. Put a sheet of filo pastry on a work surface and brush all over with melted butter. Top with another sheet of filo pastry and brush with more butter. Add a quarter of the bean mixture in a line along the long edge, then roll up into a cylinder, brushing with more butter as you roll.

4. Wind the filo tube carefully into a coil and place it on the lined baking sheet. If any cracks appear, you can just patch them up with a little extra filo pastry brushed with butter.

5. Repeat the steps above three times more, coiling each filo cylinder around the previous one to make the outer rings of the spiral. Brush the completed pie with any leftover butter and scatter over the mixed seeds. Transfer to the oven and bake for about 50 minutes, or until deep golden brown.

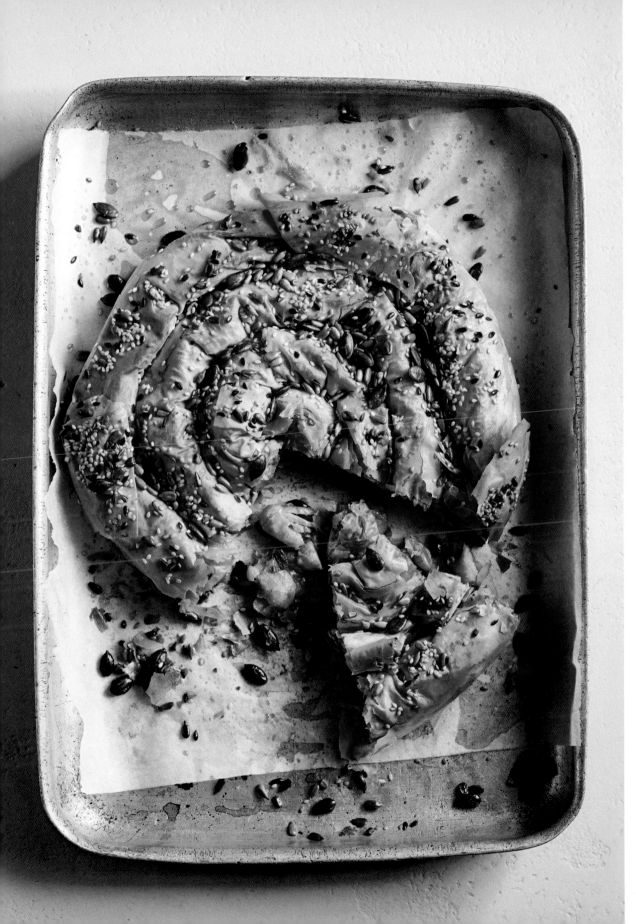

Black Lentils with Apple Cider Vinegar Pickled Pink Onions + Watercress

SERVES 2
(WITH LEFTOVERS)

Plant Diversity
Score: 5

1 tbsp vegetable oil

1 red onion, thinly sliced

1 tbsp mustard seeds

1 tsp mild chilli powder

1 tsp cumin seeds

½ tsp ground turmeric

1 tbsp tomato purée

150g (5oz/¾ cup) dried beluga lentils

1.25 litres (42fl oz/5 cups) vegetable stock

40g (1½oz) watercress leaves

Salt, to taste

FOR THE PICKLED ONIONS

1 red onion, thinly sliced

2 tbsp apple cider vinegar

1 tsp sugar

Pinch of salt

This recipe has a kind of retro appeal; the black lentils against the vivid emerald hues of watercress and shocking pink onions reminds me of an art installation from the early nineties. Unlike an art installation, however, this dish tastes great and freezes very well too. Use whichever dried lentils you prefer; the recipe will work well whatever you choose.

—

1. First prepare the pickled onions. Combine the red onion with the vinegar, sugar and salt and rub gently with your hands to help the onions take on a pink hue. Set aside for at least 15 minutes to allow the flavours to develop.

2. Heat a large saucepan over a medium heat. Add the oil and sliced onion to the pan and fry for 10 minutes until soft and starting to turn golden brown at the edges. Now add the mustard seeds, chilli powder, cumin seeds, turmeric and tomato purée, stirring well to combine. Ensure the spices don't catch – if they are looking that way, add a few splashes of water.

3. After a minute or so, when the spices have released their aroma, add the lentils and stock to the pan. Bring the mixture to the boil and then simmer over a medium heat for 1 hour. Stir the mixture occasionally, squashing some of the lentils against the side of the pan to help create a creamy lentil sauce. Season the lentils with salt to taste (bear in mind that some vegetable stocks already have added salt, so you may not need much).

4. Serve the cooked lentils with the pickled onion and watercress on the side. Rice, grains, flatbreads, chapattis or parathas would make fantastic sides.

the kitchen prescription

Apple cider vinegar

+ Apple cider vinegar has an elixir-like reputation; however, while many of its reputed benefits are true, many are exaggerations or false.

+ Filtered clear apple cider vinegar is different to unfiltered cloudy apple cider vinegar, which contains proteins, enzymes and probiotic bacteria, often referred to as 'the mother'.

+ There is some limited evidence that apple cider vinegar might help with blood sugar control and very limited evidence that it may help boost weight loss.

+ Drinking it neat may damage dental enamel and cause irritation to the oesophagus.

Freekeh with Tomatoes, Roast Peppers + Anchovies

SERVES 4

Plant Diversity
Score: 5

1 x 50g (2oz) tin anchovies in extra-virgin olive oil

1 medium onion, thinly sliced (can be frozen)

2 garlic cloves, thinly sliced

1 tsp chilli flakes

½ tsp dried oregano (or 1 sprig of fresh thyme)

1 x 400g (14oz) tin cherry tomatoes

150g (5oz) dried freekeh

150g (5oz) roasted peppers from a jar

200g (7oz) cherry tomatoes, halved

Drizzle of extra-virgin olive oil

Handful of basil leaves (optional)

No one likes the taste of uncooked tinned tomatoes straight from the tin. However, when seasoned, spiced and combined with a grain like freekeh, their acidity, sweetness and smooth-cooked texture develops beautifully in the pot. I rarely use tinned tomatoes in isolation; for me the combination of fresh and tinned tomatoes works best in almost any recipe. For this dish, tinned anchovies and both tinned and fresh tomatoes spruce up the freekeh, making this speedy, hearty storecupboard dinner a real winner.

—

1. Place a heavy-based (preferably cast-iron) pan over a medium heat. Drain the oil from the tinned anchovies straight into the pan, then add the onion and sweat for 5–7 minutes until soft and starting to turn golden brown. Now add the anchovies, garlic, chilli flakes and oregano. Stir well to combine and melt the anchovies down into the onions – make sure the mixture does not catch. Add the tinned cherry tomatoes, followed by the freekeh. Stir well to combine.

2. Fill the tomato tin twice with kettle-hot water and add to the pan. Bring to the boil, place the lid on the pan and turn the heat down to low. Simmer for about 35 minutes until the freekeh has cooked through and most of the water has been absorbed by the grains; stir every so often to ensure the grains don't catch. (Freekeh varies in the amount of water it needs to cook; older varieties may need a little more water, so add more if the mixture looks dry and the freekeh is still chewy.)

3. Roughly chop the peppers from the jar and drop these into the freekeh along with the halved cherry tomatoes. Cook through for just 2 minutes, allowing the fresh tomatoes to warm through. Serve the freekeh with a drizzle of extra-virgin olive oil and strew with a few basil leaves, if you have them to hand.

the kitchen prescription

Freekeh

+ Freekeh has a beautiful nutty, rich, almost smoke-tinged flavour. It is a fibre-dense, green coloured grain made from roasting durum wheat. It's particularly popular in Palestinian households.

+ I used dried (cracked) freekeh instead of wholegrain to save cooking time.

+ Use one part freekeh to three parts water as a rule of thumb when preparing it. It should remain slightly firm and chewy.

+ You can use freekeh in any other recipe that calls for whole grains, such as bulgur wheat, farro, rice etc.

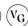

Chickpea, Fenugreek + Okra Curry

SERVES 4

Plant Diversity
Score: 7
Bonus Score: 1

For those wishing to diversify their repertoire of frozen produce, I would encourage a trip to your local Asian or Middle Eastern food store to buy frozen fenugreek leaves, also known as methi. They have a slightly bitter, earthy taste that ends with an almost maple syrup tone. Fenugreek pairs well with potatoes, chicken and – in this recipe – fibre-dense chickpeas and creamy coconut milk. Swap the frozen fenugreek leaves for frozen spinach or frozen okra if you prefer.

—

2 tbsp extra-virgin olive oil

1 white onion, thinly sliced

2 garlic cloves, grated

1 tsp ground turmeric

1 tsp chilli powder

½ tsp garam masala

2 x 400g (14oz) tins chickpeas

1 x 400ml (14fl oz) tin full-fat organic coconut milk

100g (3½oz) frozen fenugreek leaves

150g (5oz) okra, diced into 2.5cm (1in) rounds

TO SERVE

Brown or wild rice

Wedges of lemon

1. Heat the olive oil in a saucepan over a medium heat. Add the onion and fry for 6–7 minutes, then add the garlic and cook for a further 3 minutes until the onion is golden brown. Add the turmeric, chilli powder and garam masala and stir well, allowing the spices to release their aromas. Make sure that the spices do not burn and catch by controlling the heat of the pan, or by adding a few splashes of water.

2. Drain the chickpeas and add them to the onions along with the coconut milk. Bring to a simmer and cook for 5 minutes, then add the fenugreek leaves and okra. Braise the mixture for a further 10–15 minutes over a medium heat. Serve with rice and wedges of lemon for an extra citrus tang.

the kitchen prescription

Fenugreek (Trigonella foenum-graecum)

+ Fenugreek is thought to enhance breast milk production.

+ Some preliminary studies suggest that it can boost testosterone levels and libido in men.

+ There is some early evidence to suggest that fenugreek has a role in helping diabetic patients control their blood sugar.

+ Some report a slightly tangy body odour after eating fenugreek, so maybe don't eat it on a first date!

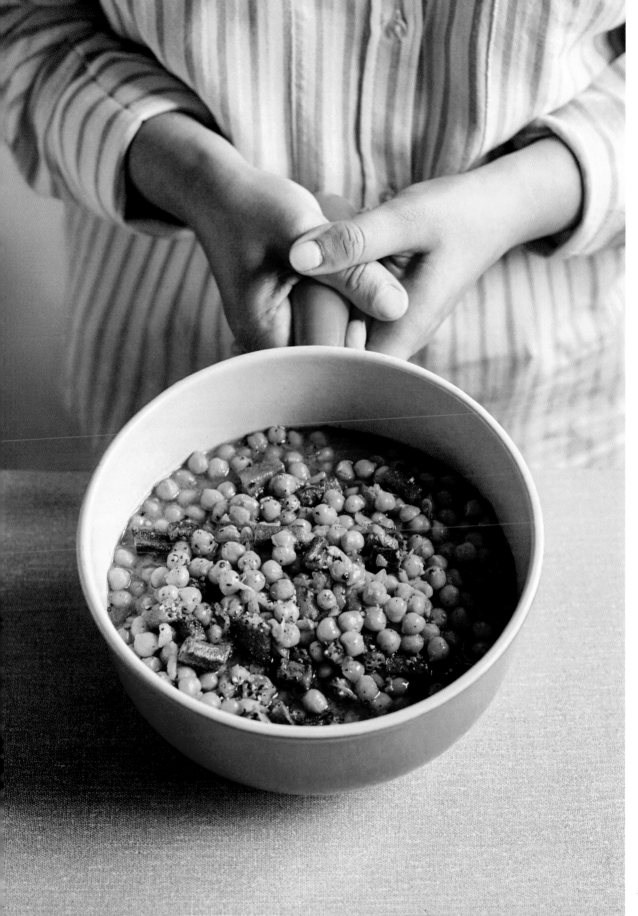

Old Ma's Khichri

SERVES 4 GENEROUSLY

Plant Diversity
Score: 5.25
Bonus Score: 0.25

Khichri is a soft lentil and rice dish popular throughout South Asia. The texture is almost risotto-like, but the chana dal gives the dish a little added bite as it doesn't break down quite as quickly as the other lentils. The addition of quinoa and turmeric gives the dish a gut-friendly, anti-inflammatory, fibre-filled boost, while the spiced garlic and oil infusion fills the air with an irresistible allium aroma.

You can serve this dish with Indian pickles, but as these are often quite heavily salted I prefer to serve this with just wedges of lemon, and the occasional poppadum.

—

25g (1oz) chana dal

25g (1oz) red lentils

25g (1oz) brown lentils

25g (1oz) quinoa

100g (3½oz/½ cup) basmati rice

1 tsp ground turmeric

1.25 litres (42fl oz/5 cups) kettle-hot water

Salt, to taste

FOR THE TADKA

2 tbsp ghee or vegetable oil

3 garlic cloves, thinly sliced

1–2 fresh red or green chillies

1 tsp cumin seeds

6 curry leaves, frozen or dried (optional)

12 twists of black pepper

1. Place the chana dal, red lentils, brown lentils, quinoa, rice, turmeric and hot water in a saucepan and bring to the boil. Simmer over a medium heat, uncovered, for 30–40 minutes, stirring every so often to ensure nothing sticks to the base of the pan. The end result will be a dish with a soupy, risotto-like consistency. Season with salt to taste.

2. While the dal is cooking, make the tadka. Heat the ghee or vegetable oil in a frying pan until hot but not quite smoking. Add the garlic, chillies, cumin seeds, curry leaves (if using) and black pepper and fry until the garlic cloves are golden. Carefully pour the hot flavoured oil over the prepared khichri.

Stuffed Potato Flatbreads + Mustard Greens

MAKES 2

Plant Diversity
Score: 6

Made completely from storecupboard ingredients (even the potatoes are tinned), this is the kind of dish made for a weekend, where you can relax and play around with the dough without having to rush. The end result is a mellow, spiced potato filling in a crisp, buttery flatbread layer. Mustard greens are part of the brassica family. I sometimes buy them fresh, but the tinned varieties are also very tasty, although the bitter, peppery taste is an acquired one. They are thought to contain a hefty dose of vitamin K, which has a role in blood clotting, and vitamin C, which has a role in boosting immunity. Use a tin of chopped spinach if you can't get tinned mustard greens.

—

FOR THE FLATBREADS

100g (3½oz/scant 1 cup) plain flour, plus extra for dusting

100g (3½oz/scant 1 cup) chickpea flour

1 tbsp vegetable oil, plus extra for frying

Pinch of salt

FOR THE FILLING

300g (10oz) tinned new potatoes (drained weight 165g/6oz)

1 tsp chilli powder

½ tsp cumin seeds

1 tsp curry powder

½ tsp nigella seeds

Handful of finely chopped coriander

FOR THE MUSTARD GREENS

2 tbsp vegetable oil or ghee

1 onion, thinly sliced

2 garlic cloves, thinly sliced

1 tsp cumin seeds

1 tsp mustard seeds

1 tsp chilli powder

½ tsp ground turmeric

500g (1lb 2oz) tinned mustard greens

1. Start by preparing the dough. Put both flours, the vegetable oil and salt in a large bowl and add just enough water to form a soft, pliable dough. Knead by hand for 5 minutes, then divide the dough into two, roll each piece into ball and return to the bowl. Cover the bowl with a cloth or clingfilm and set aside for 15 minutes.

2. Meanwhile, put the ingredients for the filling into a bowl and mash thoroughly with a fork so that the ingredients are well combined.

3. Take a piece of the dough, roll it into a perfect round ball between your hands and place it on a well-floured worktop. Use a rolling pin to roll the dough out to a circle about 20cm (8in) in diameter. Pile half of the filling into the centre of the dough circle and bring the sides of the dough up, pinching them at the top to seal in the filling. Turn the stuffed dough over so that the pinched side is face down. Gently roll the stuffed dough out again to a circle about 20cm (8in) in diameter and 3mm (⅛in) thick. Don't worry if small bits of the stuffing start showing through – this is expected and adds to the final effect. Repeat with the other piece of dough to make a second flatbread.

4. To cook the flatbreads, drizzle some extra vegetable oil into a non-stick frying pan set over a medium heat. Transfer a flatbread from the work surface to the pan and fry for 2–3 minutes each side. It should be golden and crisp. Repeat with the second flatbread.

5. To make the mustard greens, put the vegetable oil or ghee into a pan and place it over a medium heat. When the oil is hot, add the onion and fry for 3–4 minutes until it starts turning golden brown. At this point add the garlic, followed a minute or two later by the cumin seeds, mustard seeds, chilli powder and turmeric. When the spices start releasing their aromas add the mustard greens and half a mug of kettle-hot water. Stir well and simmer gently for 10 minutes or so. Serve alongside the potato flatbreads.

DINNER

Your gut-friendly supper

Dinner is a sacred time. This hallowed time starts not when we all sit at the table and eat, but when I step foot into my kitchen. I find solace in the clink of my pots and pans, the hiss of my hob and the stability of my knife. Nothing tempers a bad mood like chopping through herbs and nuts. Nothing soothes anger like playing with the fire of chilli heat. I believe that I am a better version of myself because I cook; I hope that you too can frame your time in the kitchen as less of a chore and more of an opportunity for self-reflection.

Having said this, I am also a realist. I'd love to spend 2 hours in the kitchen every evening having 'me time' but nobody, let alone me, has the time, energy or will to cook *MasterChef*-y meals daily. I have squabbling children, wet nappies and frequent iPad malfunctions that need my attention. Dinner has to be functional; it must feed my entire family's appetite, cater for the individual preferences and health requirements of every member, while at the same time reflecting my desire to sustain my family's gut health.

These are my key tips on how you can fit gut-healthy cooking into your busy lifestyle and start viewing the kitchen as a restorative space:

+ **Find gut-healthy recipes that you know will not take more than 20–30 minutes** to prepare and have a bank of these recipes to hand (either mentally, or in a folder). There are literally thousands to choose from on the internet, in cookery books, passed down by word of mouth, or even ones that you've made up. The dinner recipes in this chapter are plant-powered, fibre-filled and designed to feed your inner community of gut microbiota, while also being easy to prepare with minimal prep or clean-up.

+ **Make a meal plan.** I admit I am a serial meal planner. I select the recipes I will be making a few days in advance and tailor my shopping list accordingly.

+ **Buy ingredients that will make your cooking easier** (and therefore more enjoyable). Spice blends, pastes and condiments will add instant flavour. Use shortcuts like ready-made pizza bases, as in my version of **Primavera Pizza** on **page 162**, or ready-made fish fingers – see my recipe for **Good Gut Tacos** on **page 168**. Don't hesitate to buy ginger and garlic paste instead of spending ages peeling and pounding your own.

+ **Be kind to yourself.** If, on occasion you still feel like getting a takeaway, or have periods where you don't wish to cook, that's completely fine. This does not equate to failure. You don't need to deny yourself the pleasure of an occasional treat; it is about the bigger picture, changing the overall pattern of how you eat to one that is gut-healthy over the course of a lifetime. That said, if it's speed you're after, cooking some of the recipes in this chapter will take less time than ordering a takeaway and getting it delivered. And with practice you will get faster and faster.

+ **Make diaries or notes** of how long you have been cooking your dinners and what health benefits you are starting to notice. After about three days you may notice improved stool consistency and energy levels; after three weeks you may notice improved skin and sleep; and after three months or more you may notice weight loss and a reduction in weight-related and lifestyle-related health issues.

I have intentionally included lots of vegetarian recipes in this chapter as it is my belief that to optimise gut health, we need to increase the ratio of how many nights a week we choose vegetarian options. I still cook chicken and fish for dinner, but most definitely not every single night.

Tips for gut-healthy dinners with children

1. I have often found real success and opportunities to bond with my children by including them in meal planning discussions. It isn't always easy to maintain control of the situation with two opinionated boys whose idea of meal planning is whether to have pasta with cheese or cheese with pasta... Nonetheless, I have found that making decisions on what is for dinner each week, putting together a list and then going shopping for gut-healthy ingredients together has, in many ways, helped my children ignite their love of and interest in food.

2. It's also fun to include them. They laugh when I tell them the botanical names of fruits and vegetables, and I laugh when they tell me how ice cream grows on trees. I try (and often fail) to educate them about the origin of the foods they pick up (albeit in a supermarket and not a farm), because I want them to appreciate the incredible efforts that other people go to so that we can have food on our table.

3. Involving my children in meal planning means that I can not only develop their palates, but also bond with them over a shared interest. I got them to name different meal days, so now Vegnesday (Vegetarian Wednesday) and Tuber Tuesday (the root vegetable, not the musical instrument) are regular calendar events, and whenever there are brassicas on the menu, the person who farts is forgiven for their 'brassica belly'.

Aubergine Pitta Pockets

SERVES 4

Plant Diversity
Score: 8
Bonus Score: 1

There will be dishes in your repertoire which are inherently gut-healthy, but perhaps you never realised just how healthy they were until you took a closer look at the ingredients. This aubergine pitta pocket is packed full of gut-friendly white cabbage, a wonderful prebiotic brassica. I find it to be an extremely satisfying alternative to burgers for dinner; the salty aubergines against the creaminess of soft-boiled eggs, dense earthiness of tahini and the light citrus zest of crunchy salad is a real dinnertime treat.

—

1 aubergine, sliced into 1cm (½in) thick rounds

4 tbsp extra-virgin olive oil

4 wholewheat pitta breads

4 heaped tsp tahini

4 soft-boiled eggs (6-minute boil), halved

4 tbsp mango chutney (optional)

FOR THE SALAD

150g (5oz) white cabbage, thinly sliced

½ red onion, thinly sliced

220g (8oz) cherry tomatoes, halved

Juice of ½ lemon

½ cucumber, thinly sliced

Handful of roughly chopped parsley and mint

Handful of pomegranate seeds (optional)

1 tbsp extra-virgin olive oil

1 tsp sumac

Salt, to taste

1. Brush the aubergine slices on both sides with the olive oil and sprinkle with salt. Place a griddle pan over a high heat; when it is really hot add the aubergines – they take 3–4 minutes on each side to leave griddle marks and to cook through completely.

2. Mix together all the ingredients for the salad in a bowl, tossing everything together well to combine.

3. Toast your pitta breads in the toaster for a few minutes. Gently open them up with a sharp knife. Stuff the pitta pocket in this order: a teaspoon of tahini at the base, followed by a large handful of salad, then the aubergine slices, then a soft-boiled egg at the top. Drizzled with the mango chutney (if using) and consume greedily.

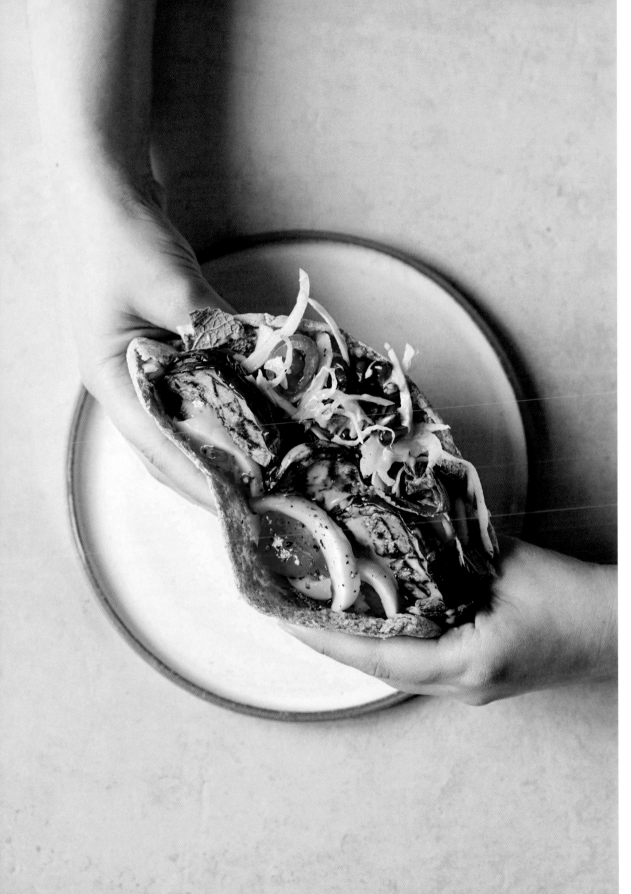

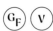

Trio of Baked Sweet Potatoes

SERVES 2

Plant Diversity
Score: 3; 2.5; 4.25

2 medium sweet potatoes

2 tsp olive oil

Pinch of flaky sea salt

Sweet potato recipes are virtually endless; it really is one of the most versatile root vegetables. My favourite way of eating sweet potato is baked, as the flesh becomes naturally buttery, caramel sweet and pillow soft. I have offered a few gut-healthy toppings for sweet potatoes here, but by all means use the same toppings on a normal baked potato if you wish. Each topping recipe make enough for 2 sweet potatoes, so scale up if you have more hungry diners.

Topping 1: Roasted Pepper + Tahini Mascarpone Crème

125g (4oz) mascarpone or cream cheese, at room temperature

2 tbsp tahini

150g (5oz) jarred roasted red peppers, finely chopped

50g (2oz) toasted walnuts, roughly chopped (or other nuts of your choice)

1 tbsp finely chopped dill (or other herb of your choice)

Salt, to taste

Mix the mascarpone and tahini in a bowl and season with salt to taste. Spread this tahini mascarpone crème on to the open sweet potatoes. Top with the jarred peppers, walnuts and dill.

Topping 2: Labneh, Cheddar + Chilli

4 tbsp labneh or thick Greek yoghurt

75g (2¾oz) grated mature Cheddar cheese

Pinch of salt

½–1 tsp chilli flakes

1 tbsp finely chopped chives

50g (2oz) rocket leaves

Combine the labneh with the Cheddar and salt and mix well. Spread this mixture over the opened sweet potatoes and sprinkle over the chilli flakes. Transfer to a hot grill for 4–5 minutes to melt the cheese. Sprinkle over the chives and serve with the rocket leaves alongside.

Topping 3: Chickpea, Chermoula + Feta

200g (7oz) tinned chickpeas

25g (1oz) melted butter

2 heaped tbsp olive, seed and pistachio chermoula (page 180)

50g (2oz) crumbled feta cheese

Salt, to taste

Combine the chickpeas with the melted butter in a small saucepan. Allow the chickpeas to heat through – this takes about 5 minutes. Smash the chickpeas slightly with the back of a wooden spoon. Add the chermoula to the chickpeas and season with salt to taste. Spoon the chickpeas on to the open sweet potatoes and top with the crumbled feta. If you don't have time to make the chermoula, use pesto instead.

the kitchen prescription

Sweet potato (Ipomoea batatas L.)

+ Do not discard the skin of your sweet potato – there's lots of gut-friendly fibre in the skin.

+ Purple sweet potatoes are rich in an antioxidant called anthocyanin, thought to be cardioprotective.

+ Sweet potatoes are a rich source of beta-carotene, which our body uses to make vitamin A, a necessary nutrient for healthy night vision.

+ Cooking sweet potatoes does decrease their beta-carotene content, but increases their vitamin C content.

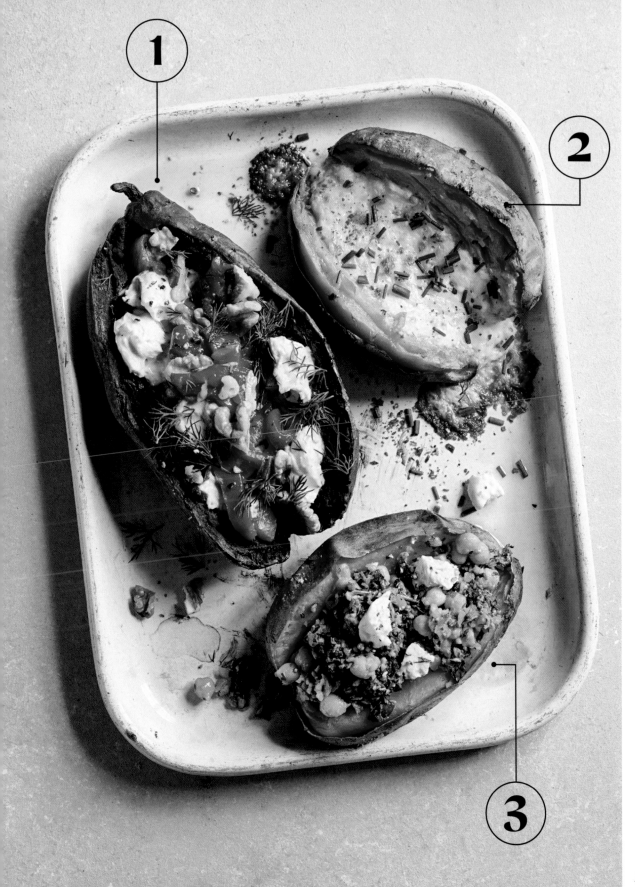

Vibrant Green Paneer

SERVES 4

Plant Diversity
Score: 5

Paneer, a protein-rich cheese made from milk curds, tastes quite bland on its own but is a wonderful sponge for the bold flavours we will introduce in this recipe. It is a great meat-free alternative to chicken for dinner, but this marinade would also work very well on chicken or juicy prawns, if you prefer.

—

500g (1lb 2oz) block of paneer

½ red onion, thinly sliced

1 tomato, thinly sliced

50g (2oz) spinach leaves

1 tbsp lemon juice

½ tsp red chilli powder (optional)

200g (7oz) live natural yoghurt

4 wholewheat flatbreads/ wraps/roti/naan

Salt, to taste

FOR THE MARINADE

3 garlic cloves

1 tsp cumin seeds

1 tsp coriander seeds

1 tsp chilli flakes

Juice of ½ lemon

2 tbsp extra-virgin olive oil

100g (3½oz) baby-leaf spinach

Handful of coriander leaves

Salt, to taste

1. Place all the ingredients for the marinade in a blender and blitz to a smooth purée.

2. Cut the paneer into fish finger-shaped pieces and place them in a bowl. Pour two-thirds of the marinade over the paneer, keeping the remaining third aside. Stir the marinade into the paneer so that it is coated all over.

3. Place a griddle pan over a medium-high heat. Add the paneer to the griddle pan and cook for about 1–2 minutes on each side. You should have satisfying dark griddle marks on the paneer.

4. Combine the onion, tomato, spinach leaves, lemon juice and chilli powder to make a quick salad. Season with salt to taste. Take the remaining marinade and swirl it into the yoghurt to create a vivid green dip. Toast your flatbreads in the grill or toaster.

5. To serve ,top the flatbreads with a generous spoonful of the yoghurt dip, followed by the griddled paneer and the salad. Serve immediately.

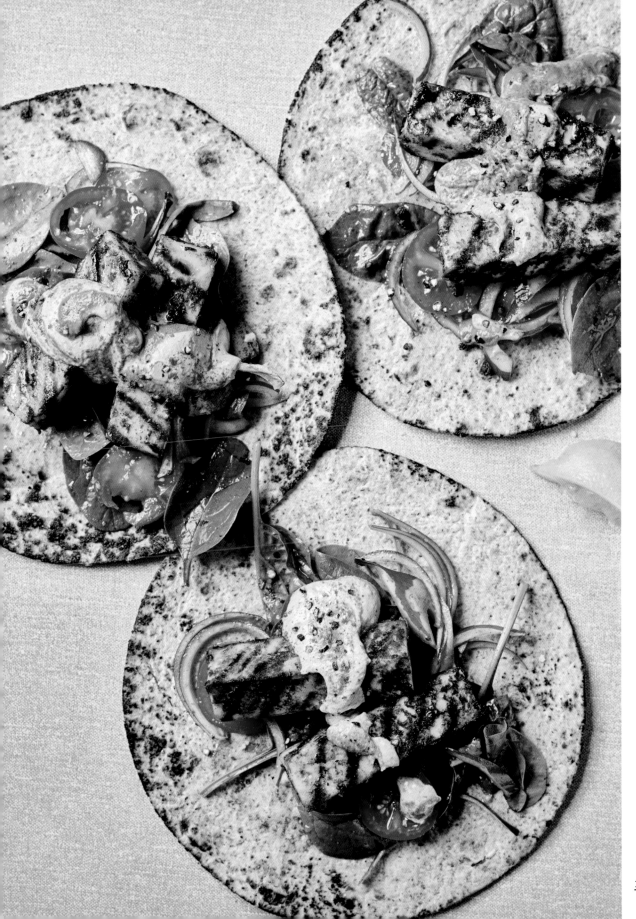

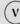

Speedy Midweek Vegetable Ratatouille

SERVES 4

Plant Diversity
Score: 5.25
Bonus Score: 1

An easily adaptable dish depending on what leftover vegetables you have lurking in the fridge. I keep the vegetables quite chunky, for texture and ease. When they are in season I use sweet, ripe fresh tomatoes to produce a lighter, brighter and less wet ratatouille but you could also use a tin of good-quality chopped tomatoes. Perfect with some warm seedy bread and garlic butter.

—

3 tbsp extra-virgin olive oil

2 portobello mushrooms, sliced 1cm (½in) thick

2 tsp garlic paste

2 courgettes, halved and chopped into thick batons

1 large red pepper, cut into thick chunks

1 tsp chilli flakes

1 tsp dried thyme or oregano

3 ripe tomatoes, roughly chopped

2 tbsp finely chopped parsley

Salt, to taste

BONUS GUT-FRIENDLY ADDITIONS

Chunks of aubergine, red onion or carrots, added with the mushrooms

1. Drizzle the olive oil into a large, shallow, cast-iron dish and place over a medium heat. When the oil is hot but not smoking, add the mushrooms (and bonus gut-friendly additions, if using) and fry for 5 minutes until they turn a deep brown colour. Add the garlic to the fried mushrooms; after a minute or two, add the courgettes, red pepper, chilli flakes and thyme. Stir everything together to combine. Allow the vegetables to cook for about 10 minutes, stirring every so often to prevent catching.

2. Once the vegetables have started to caramelise and soften, add the tomatoes and 200ml (7fl oz/generous ¾ cup) water to the pan. Cover with a lid and simmer for a further 10 minutes before serving, sprinkled with the chopped parsley.

Summery Five Veg Rice with Mackerel + Tomato Relish

SERVES 4

Plant Diversity
Score: 7.25
Bonus Score: 0.25

In this recipe I use poha, a pressed, dehydrated rice which takes minutes to prepare and is a great little time-saving addition to your pantry. You could, of course, use 500g (1lb 2oz) of any pre-cooked rice instead, but there is something totally magical about watching the poha flakes come to life in the wok. To make this dish gut-friendly I have used five different vegetables: forget worrying about five a day when you can have five in one dish!

—

FOR THE POHA RICE

3 tbsp vegetable oil

1 red onion, thinly sliced

1 tsp black mustard seeds

8 curry leaves (optional)

1 tsp cumin seeds

½–1 tsp chilli flakes

1 level tsp ground turmeric

1 courgette, cut into 1cm (½in) dice

100g (3½oz) frozen broad beans or peas, defrosted

100g (3½oz) green beans, cut into 1–2cm (½–¾in) pieces

250g (9oz) pressed rice (poha/pawa rice)

2 fillets of smoked mackerel

Handful of chopped coriander

Salt, to taste

FOR THE RELISH

1 ripe tomato, roughly chopped

1 green chilli, roughly chopped

Juice of 1 lemon

Handful of fresh coriander

½ tsp sugar

1. Add the vegetable oil to a wok and fry the red onion over a medium heat. When the onion is barely golden (after about 3 minutes), add the mustard seeds, curry leaves (if using), cumin seeds, chilli flakes and turmeric. Stir well to make sure that none of the spices catch. Add the courgette, broad beans (or peas) and green beans and stir well so that everything is coated evenly in the spices.

2. To prepare the pressed rice, pour warm water into a large bowl. Drop the pressed rice into the warm water and leave for 15 seconds, then drain in a sieve. Drop the wet rice immediately into the wok with the prepared vegetables and stir well. Within 1–2 minutes the rice will have rehydrated completely. Flake in the mackerel, discarding the skin. Season with salt to taste and garnish with plenty of chopped coriander.

3. Combine all the ingredients for the relish together to form a chunky relish. Season with salt to taste and serve alongside the vegetable rice.

Chilli Salmon + Greens

SERVES 4

Plant Diversity
Score: 5

This recipe is my gut-friendly alternative to a Chinese takeaway. It takes less time to cook and get it on the table than ordering from your local and is so much healthier than any takeaway I have ever bought. Pack yours with as many vegetables as you have to hand: Chinese cabbage, peas, Tenderstem broccoli or carrots would make great additions here. I serve this with vermicelli noodles or leftover rice, starches which do a great job of soaking up all the flavoursome juices. But I often have it just as is: no sides, just pink-fleshed, omega-3-rich, flaky salmon against the satisfying crunch of the medley of vegetables.

—

2 pak choi, washed and stems trimmed

200g (7oz) green beans, trimmed

100g (3½oz) sugar snap peas

4 salmon fillets, skin removed

4 spring onions, sliced into thin strips

FOR THE MARINADE

4 tsp Lao Gan Ma crispy chillies in oil (or any chilli oil)

1 level tbsp sesame oil

1 tbsp soy sauce

1 tsp garlic paste

1 tsp ginger paste

1. Preheat the oven to 180°C fan/200°C/gas mark 6.

2. Lay out 4 large pieces of foil on your work surface, shiny side down, dull side up. If your foil is not very strong, use two sheets instead of one. Divide the vegetables equally across the 4 pieces of foil, placing them in a heap in the centre of each piece. Lay a salmon fillet on top of each pile of vegetables and finally top with the spring onions.

3. Mix together all the ingredients for the marinade in a small bowl. Spoon the marinade equally over the 4 pieces of salmon. Now bring the edges of the foil together loosely and then secure the parcel tightly by crimping the opposing edges together. It doesn't really matter what the parcels looks like, just that it they are all sealed tight. Transfer the 4 parcels carefully to a baking tray and bake in the oven for 20 minutes. Serve each parcel to be opened at the table.

NOTE

For a meat-free alternative, try a 150g (5oz) chunk of firm tofu instead of salmon.

---

the kitchen prescription

Pak choi, aka bok choy or pok choi (Brassica rapa subsp. chinensis)

+ A variety of Chinese cabbage, pak choi is a cruciferous vegetable in the same family as kale, Brussels sprouts and broccoli. It is the most widely eaten brassica in China, and is a good source of vitamins C, A and K and fibre.

+ Its dark, velvety leaves are thought to benefit the functioning of the thyroid gland (a butterfly-shaped gland in the neck that produces essential hormones) and may be beneficial for heart and bone health.

+ There are compelling links now being drawn between the consumption of leafy greens like pak choi and a reduced risk of developing certain cancers.

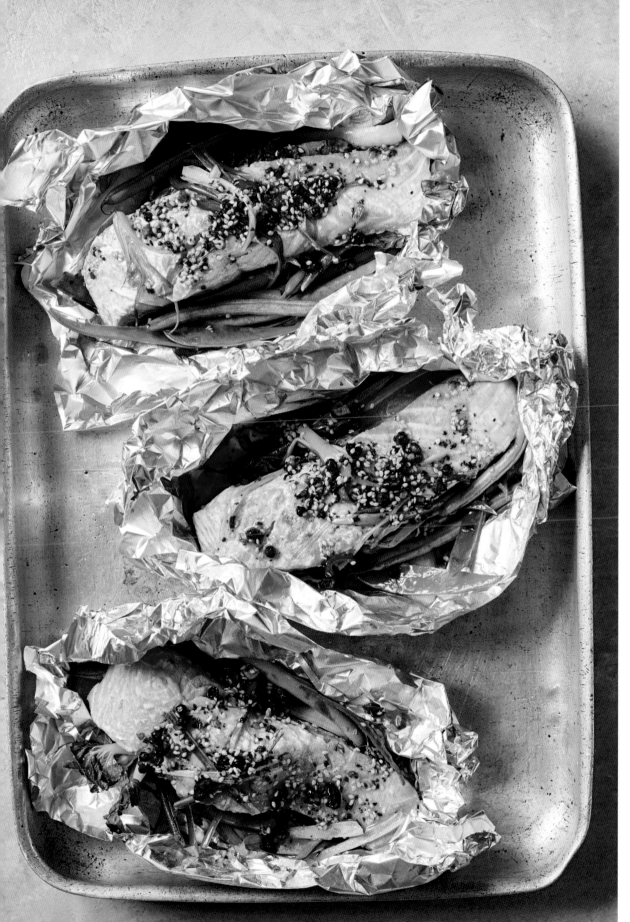

Golden Sesame Chicken with Japanese-style Sesame Salad + Sauce

SERVES 4

Plant Diversity
Score: 5.75

Your midweek dose of gut love starts and ends with this flavour explosion. For extra flavour (and as a time-saving strategy), make the mince mixture and dipping sauce the night before. I use ready-cooked jasmine rice that comes in a microwaveable packet as well as pre-prepared ginger and garlic pastes; your time is precious too, so take advantage of these shortcuts.

—

400g (14oz) cooked jasmine rice (about 2 microwaveable pouches)

FOR THE CHICKEN

500g (1lb 2oz) minced chicken

2 tsp red chilli paste

1 heaped tsp garlic paste

1 heaped tsp ginger paste

4 spring onions, thinly sliced

100g (3½oz/⅔ cup) sesame seeds (white, black or both)

1 tbsp vegetable oil

Salt, to taste

FOR THE SESAME SAUCE

3 tbsp tahini

4 tbsp mayonnaise

1 tbsp rice vinegar

2 tsp sesame oil

2 tbsp soy sauce

1 tsp sugar

FOR THE SALAD

½ mooli or 8–10 pink radishes, thinly sliced

1 carrot, peeled and thinly sliced

½ cucumber, thinly sliced

1 tsp sesame seeds

I tsp rice vinegar

1. In a bowl, combine the minced chicken with the red chilli, garlic and ginger pastes, the spring onions and salt to taste. Divide the chicken into 8 equal-sized portions.

2. Place the sesame seeds in a shallow dish. Heat a non-stick frying pan over a medium heat and brush the surface of the pan with the vegetable oil. Take each portion of chicken and use your hands to shape it into flat, round patty, about 1cm (½in) thick. If you rub a little oil on to the palms of your hands before doing this it makes it much easier to handle the meat.

3. Dip each chicken patty into the sesame seeds, coating both sides, then add to the frying pan. Cook in batches of two or three for about 2½ minutes on each side. Be careful to not have the pan too hot, as otherwise the sesame seeds will burn before the chicken has cooked through.

4. For the sauce, mix all the ingredients together in a small bowl to form a smooth sauce. Toss all the salad ingredients together in a large bowl and season with salt to taste.

5. Heat the rice according to the packet instructions. Serve the rice with 2 chicken patties per portion, a generous handful of salad and the dipping sauce alongside.

---

the kitchen prescription

Sesame seeds (Sesamum indicum L.)

+ These tiny oily seeds are a fantastic source of dietary fibre. They come in white, golden and black varieties.

+ Sesame seeds are full of lignans like sesamin, sesamolin and sesaminol and plant phytosterols, which seem to possess antioxidant and cholesterol-reducing properties.

+ The benefits of sesame oil are even mentioned in the ancient Hindu Vedas. It has been used for centuries as a natural treatment for skin infections.

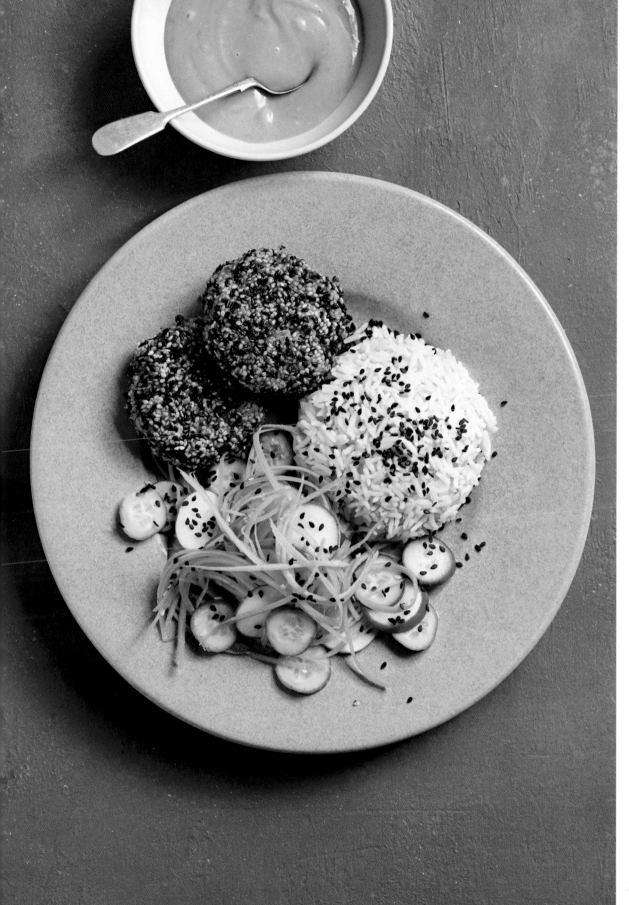

Ten-minute Gochujang Noodles

SERVES 2
(WITH LEFTOVERS)

Plant Diversity
Score: 4.5

Gochujang is a Korean fermented spice paste made from gochugaru chilli powder, glutinous rice, meju (fermented soybean powder) and yeotgireum (barley malt powder). It's well worth having in your pantry as a dinnertime flavour shortcut; you can use this stellar condiment in practically any way you like: baked on cauliflower, rippled in mayonnaise, as a seasoning to fishcakes, and so on. In this recipe, prawns and vegetables are cooked in this paste and then paired with egg noodles; it's a combination that is guaranteed to have you heading back to the wok for seconds.

NOTE

If you can't get hold of gochujang, make a cheat's version by blending 5 pitted Medjool dates, 1 tablespoon of apple cider vinegar, 1 heaped tablespoon of tomato purée, 1 heaped teaspoon of chilli flakes and 1 teaspoon of garlic granules to a smooth purée with a touch of warm water. Alternatively, use a shop-bought stir-fry sauce such as teriyaki sauce, hoisin, chow mein, black bean, or sweet and sour.

—

1 heaped tbsp gochujang paste (see Note)

1 tbsp sesame oil

2 tbsp soy sauce

1 heaped tsp ginger paste

1 heaped tsp garlic paste

3 pak choi (about 200g/7oz)

1 tbsp vegetable oil

300g (10oz) raw and peeled king prawns (or 250g/9oz tofu cubes)

100g (3½oz) white cabbage, thinly sliced

1 x 225g (8oz) tin sliced water chestnuts (about 140g/4½oz drained weight)

400g (14oz) cooked 'straight to wok' medium egg noodles

1 tbsp black or white sesame seeds

Salt, to taste

1. Start by mixing together the gochujang paste with the sesame oil, soy sauce and ginger and garlic pastes in a small bowl. Loosen the mixture with about 100ml (3½fl oz/scant ½ cup) of kettle-hot water. This is your stir-fry sauce. Season with just a little more salt to taste if you wish.

2. Slice the base of the pak choi into thin rounds; keep the leaves intact and set them aside for later. Place a wok over a high heat; when it is roaring hot, add the vegetable oil followed by the king prawns. They will turn from grey to pink in seconds. Quickly add the sliced base of the pak choi, cabbage and water chestnuts, stirring frequently. Cook for 2–3 minutes and make sure you keep the heat high to prevent the vegetables from stewing.

3. Now add the stir-fry sauce to the wok, followed a minute later by the cooked noodles and the leafy tips of the pak choi. Stir everything well to combine. If the pan looks a little dry at this stage, you can add a little more water to create a saucy consistency. It will take no more than 2–3 more minutes in the wok to cook through. Serve garnished with sesame seeds.

Middle Eastern-style Beany Quesadillas with Guacamole

SERVES 4

Plant Diversity
Score: 5

This Middle Eastern-Mexican mash-up is designed to become a family favourite. Beany, cheesy ooziness against buttery avocado and tart sumac is the definition of a dream dinner. My children ask for this dish often. Thankfully it is really easy to make.

—

FOR THE QUESADILLAS

120g (4oz) tinned sweetcorn

1 x 400g (14oz) tin mixed beans, drained

120g (4oz) grated Manchego cheese (or 150g/5oz grated Cheddar cheese)

½ tsp chilli flakes (or black pepper if your kids don't like spice)

2 tsp pomegranate molasses

1 tsp garlic granules

4 spring onions, white parts only, thinly sliced

Handful of finely chopped parsley leaves

8 tortilla wraps (corn and wheat mix), about 20cm (8in) in diameter

FOR THE GUACAMOLE

2 avocados

4 spring onions, green parts only, thinly sliced

Juice of 1 lemon

1 tsp sumac

½ tsp chilli flakes

1 tbsp extra-virgin olive oil

Handful of finely chopped parsley

Flaky sea salt

1. Combine the sweetcorn, beans, cheese, chilli flakes, pomegranate molasses, garlic granules, spring onions and parsley in a bowl. Mash together lightly with a fork to break some of the beans down a bit and mix everything together well.

2. Spread a quarter of this mixture on to a tortilla and top with another tortilla, pressing firmly to sandwich everything together. Repeat to make 4 quesadillas in total.

3. Halve and stone the avocados and use a spoon to scoop out the avocado flesh into a bowl. Add the spring onions, lemon juice, sumac, chilli flakes, olive oil and parsley to the avocado and roughly mash everything together. Season with salt to taste.

4. Heat a non-stick pan over a medium-low heat. Place a quesadilla in the pan and toast on each side for 3–4 minutes, or until golden on each side. Repeat until all the quesadillas are cooked. Cut in half with a sharp knife before serving with the guacamole.

---

the kitchen prescription

Avocado (Persea americana)

+ Numerous studies have shown that avocados are beneficial to our cardiometabolic health; they are rich in plant-based fats – up to 80 per cent of the calories in avocados come from healthy fats, similar to extra-virgin olive oil.

+ There is evidence that avocados can reduce the 'bad' (LDL) type of cholesterol in your body, and raise levels of 'good' (HDL) cholesterol.

+ Avocados are amazing, but they might be *too* amazing. The environmental impact of our society's overconsumption of avocados is significant; however, if you have them only occasionally, you can enjoy their health benefits without feeling too much like you're destroying the planet.

Kimchi + Garlic Fried Rice

SERVES 4

Plant Diversity
Score: 6.5

It's a terrible waste for leftover rice to end up in the bin. Thankfully this recipe is a great blueprint to have in your repertoire for when you've cooked too much rice. The combination of garlic, kimchi and chilli oil makes for an outstanding dish that you can rustle up in minutes. Feel free to add any other vegetables from your fridge instead of (or alongside) the suggested vegetables here. Leave out the fried eggs to keep this vegan.

—

Vegetable oil, for frying

3 garlic cloves, thinly sliced

4 spring onions, finely chopped

1 grated carrot

120g (4oz) white cabbage, finely shredded

½ green pepper, finely diced

450g (1lb) cooked and cooled rice (or use ready-cooked pouches)

100g (3½oz) frozen peas, defrosted

1 tbsp dark soy sauce

200g (7oz) kimchi, roughly chopped, plus extra to serve

4 tsp Lao Gan Ma crispy chillies in oil (or any chilli oil)

4 eggs (optional)

Salt, to taste

1. Add 2 tablespoons of vegetable oil to a frying pan or wok and crank up the heat to high. Add the garlic and spring onions and when they have started to turn golden (after just a minute or two), add the carrot, cabbage and green pepper. Ensure that the heat remains high as you want the vegetables fry quickly and caramelise, rather than stew.

2. After 2 minutes, add the rice to the frying pan along with the peas, soy sauce and chopped kimchi. Splash about 3 tablespoons of warm water into the pan. The steam will soften the rice and bring all the ingredients together. Give everything a good toss to combine and within a minute or so your fried rice will be ready. Taste and season with salt if you feel the dish needs it (the kimchi and soy sauce are already salty, so be cautious).

3. Fry the eggs in a drizzle of vegetable oil in a non-stick pan over a medium heat until the edges are crispy but the yolks are still runny. Place the rice in 4 bowls and top each one with a fried egg and a drizzle of chilli oil. Eat immediately, with some extra kimchi on the side.

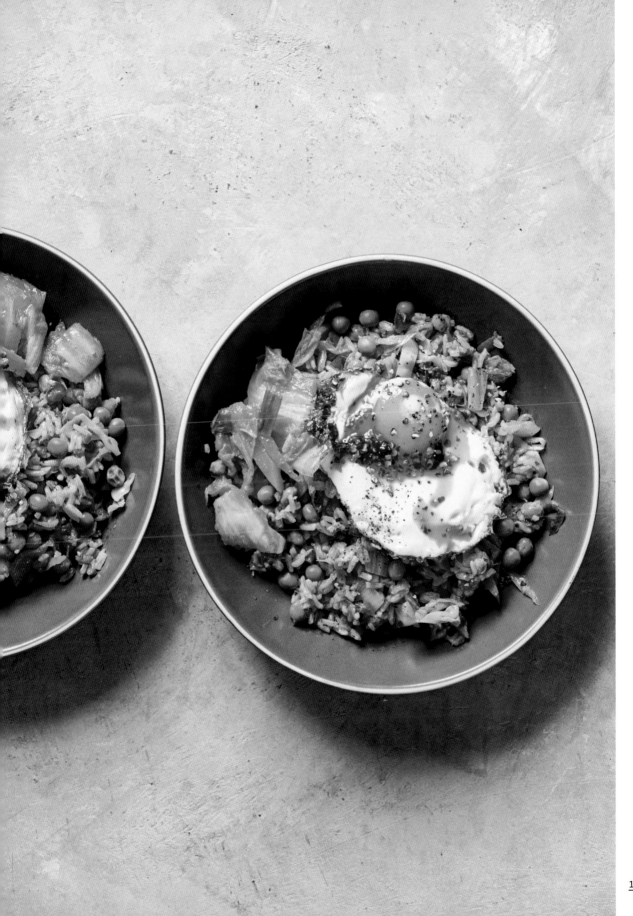

Primavera Pizza

MAKES 1 PIZZA
(SERVES 2)

Plant Diversity
Score: 5
Bonus Score: 3

A gut-friendly pizza version of the classic vegetable-laden pasta dish, guaranteed to please you and your gut. Customise according to whichever vegetable toppings you have to hand and feel free to make your own pizza dough, maybe even using khorasan or spelt flour if you are feeling adventurous. But, for a midweek meal, I must admit I often buy shop-bought pizza dough as a time-saving strategy.

—

1 tbsp extra-virgin olive oil, plus 1 tsp

400g (14oz) ready-made pizza dough (pre-rolled or ready-to-roll)

3 tbsp smooth tomato passata

½ tsp garlic paste

½ tsp dried oregano

4 sun-dried tomatoes, roughly chopped

½ courgette, thinly sliced into ribbons using a vegetable peeler

5 jarred chargrilled artichokes, roughly chopped

5 asparagus spears, sliced in half lengthways

50g (2oz) firm goats' cheese, sliced into thin rounds

½ tsp chilli flakes

2 tbsp grated Parmesan (or vegetarian hard-style Italian cheese)

1 heaped tbsp toasted pine nuts

Handful of rocket leaves

Salt, to taste

1. Preheat the oven to 200°C fan/220°C/gas mark 7. Place a sheet of baking paper on a large baking sheet and brush it with just a teaspoon of olive oil. Transfer the rolled-out pizza dough carefully on to the baking paper.

2. Mix the tomato passata with the garlic paste and oregano and then spread it over the pizza dough, leaving a 2cm (¾in) rim around the edge. Now arrange the sun-dried tomatoes, courgette ribbons, artichokes and asparagus over the tomato sauce. Scatter over the goats' cheese, season with salt and chilli flakes and drizzle over the tablespoon of olive oil. Transfer to the oven for 20–25 minutes to bake until golden and cooked through. Scatter over the Parmesan, pine nuts and rocket just before serving.

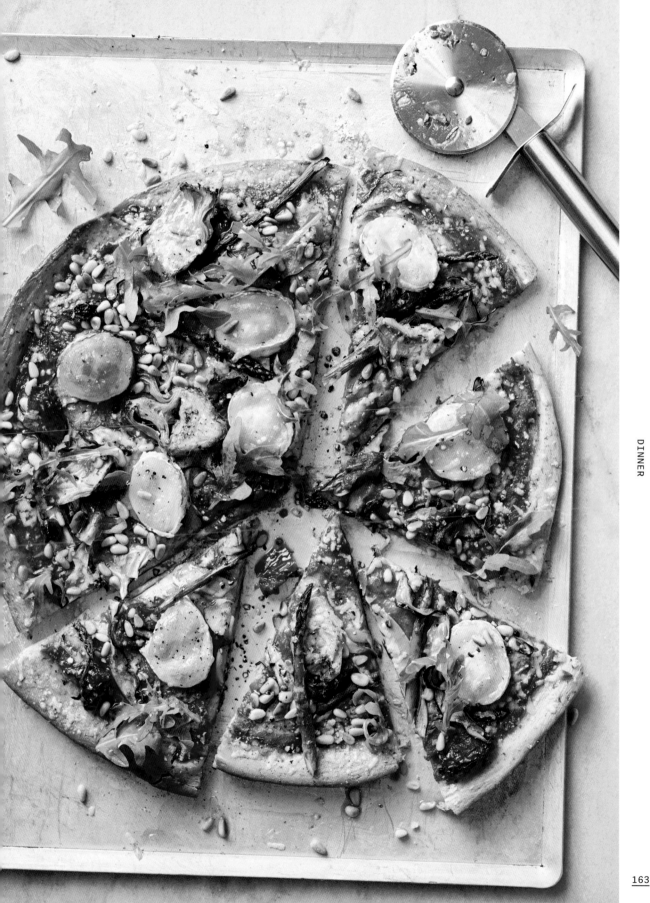

Za'atar Lasagne Verde

Plant Diversity
Score: 6.75

A very green, rustic lasagne. I love this recipe not just for how veg-packed and gut-friendly it is, but also for the fact that because there is no braising meat or stirring béchamel involved, it takes literally no time to assemble compared to a classic meat lasagne.

—

1 tbsp olive oil

3 garlic cloves, thinly sliced

6 spring onions, finely chopped

2 large courgettes, diced into small cubes

150g (5oz) cavolo nero or kale, finely chopped

150g (5oz) broccoli florets, finely chopped

125g (4oz) frozen peas

2 tbsp za'atar

500g (1lb 2oz) mascarpone

500g (1lb 2oz) ricotta cheese

100ml (3½fl oz/scant ½ cup) whole milk

150g (5oz/1½ cups) grated Parmesan cheese (or vegetarian hard-style Italian cheese)

8 sheets of fresh egg lasagne (not the dried sheets)

Salt and freshly ground black pepper

1. Preheat the oven to 180°C fan/200°C/gas mark 6.

2. Start by heating the olive oil in a large frying pan and adding the garlic. When the garlic starts to brown a little, add the spring onions, courgettes, cavolo nero, broccoli and peas. Cook them through for 3–4 minutes over a high heat to wilt the vegetables down a little and to brown off the courgettes. Sprinkle half the za'atar over the vegetables and stir well. Season generously with salt and pepper.

3. Mix the mascarpone with the ricotta and milk and whisk to form a smooth sauce. Add half the Parmesan to this mixture. You are now ready to build your lasagne in your chosen dish (I use a 30 x 20cm/12 x 8in ceramic oven dish).

4. Layer up the lasagne, starting with sheets of pasta, then vegetables, then cheese sauce and repeating until you have made 3 or 4 layers. Make sure you finish with a layer of pasta, followed by a good amount of the cheese sauce (about a third). Sprinkle the remaining Parmesan and za'atar over the top of the lasagne, then bake in the oven for 50 minutes–1 hour, or until a deep golden crust has formed.

the kitchen prescription

Za'atar

+ Za'atar is an ancient herb blend from the Middle East that is referenced in the Bible. It's made from wild thyme, oregano, marjoram, sumac, sesame seeds and salt.

+ Thought to be a robust antioxidant with some antimicrobial properties, it is also used across the Levant to help clear the respiratory tract. Although there are no formal studies to assess how good it is at this, there is a lot of anecdotal evidence for its effectiveness.

+ In Palestine, children are encouraged to have za'atar for breakfast, as people believe that it contributes to mental alertness.

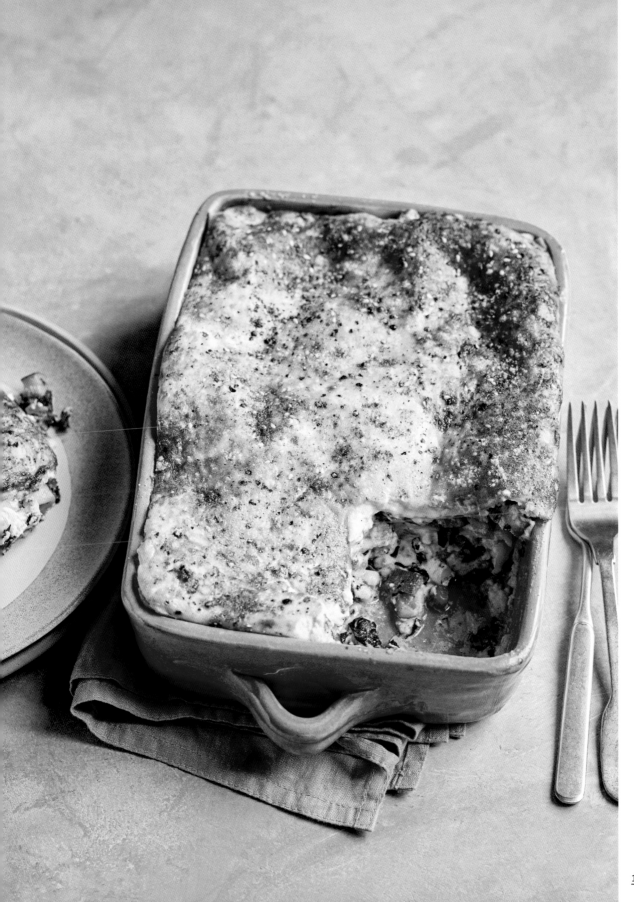

Orecchiette with Labneh, Herbs + Tomatoes

SERVES 2
(WITH LEFTOVERS)

Plant Diversity
Score: 2.5
Bonus Score: 1 or more

In my cooking I tend to treat herbs, particularly dill and parsley, like a salad leaf; I use large quantities, and chop them roughly (if at all). These herbs are so deeply flavoured that when paired with creamy probiotic labneh and pasta, they can make the most colourful dishes. In this recipe you can use any vegetable of your choice instead of tomatoes: sautéed mushrooms, peppers, aubergines, kale or spinach would also be wonderful.

—

180g (6oz) dried orecchiette (or other pasta of your choice)

300g (10oz) labneh, at room temperature (see Note)

2 garlic cloves, grated

Juice of ½–1 lemon

Large handful of finely chopped parsley

Large handful of finely chopped dill

Salt, to taste

FOR THE TOMATOES

1 tbsp olive oil, plus extra for drizzling

50g (2oz) melted butter

½ tsp dried oregano

½ tsp chilli flakes

250g (9oz) cherry tomatoes, halved

BONUS GUT-FRIENDLY ADDITIONS

Toasted pine nuts or toasted mixed seeds scattered over the tomatoes before serving

1. Bring a large saucepan of salted water to the boil and cook the orecchiette according to the packet instructions. Drain, reserving the drained pasta water.

2. Place the labneh in a large bowl and add the garlic, lemon juice, dill and parsley (reserve a little of each herb to dress the final dish). Season with salt to taste. Loosen the labneh with a few splashes of pasta water and add the drained pasta. Stir well to combine.

3. For the tomatoes, heat the olive oil and butter in a saucepan over a low-medium heat. When the butter is foaming, add the oregano and chilli flakes. Allow the spices and butter to bubble for a minute or so before adding the tomatoes. Cook the tomatoes in the butter for a minute or so, then season with salt to taste. The idea is to blister the tomatoes but not break them down.

4. Spoon the tomatoes on to the orecchiette. Drizzle with a little more olive oil and scatter with the reserved herbs, then serve immediately.

NOTE
If you can't get hold of labneh, you can make your own by straining Greek yoghurt through a cheesecloth in the fridge overnight, suspended over a bowl to catch the water that drips out of it. Or just use strained live Greek yoghurt instead.

the kitchen prescription

Labneh

+ Labneh is a nutrient-dense probiotic, rich in calcium and protein. It can be made from both cows' and goats' milk and is fermented by lactic acid bacteria, giving it a slightly sourer taste than yoghurt.

+ Due to being strained and fermented, labneh contains less lactose than other types of cheese. As a result, it is anecdotally said to be a better tolerated by those with mild lactose intolerance.

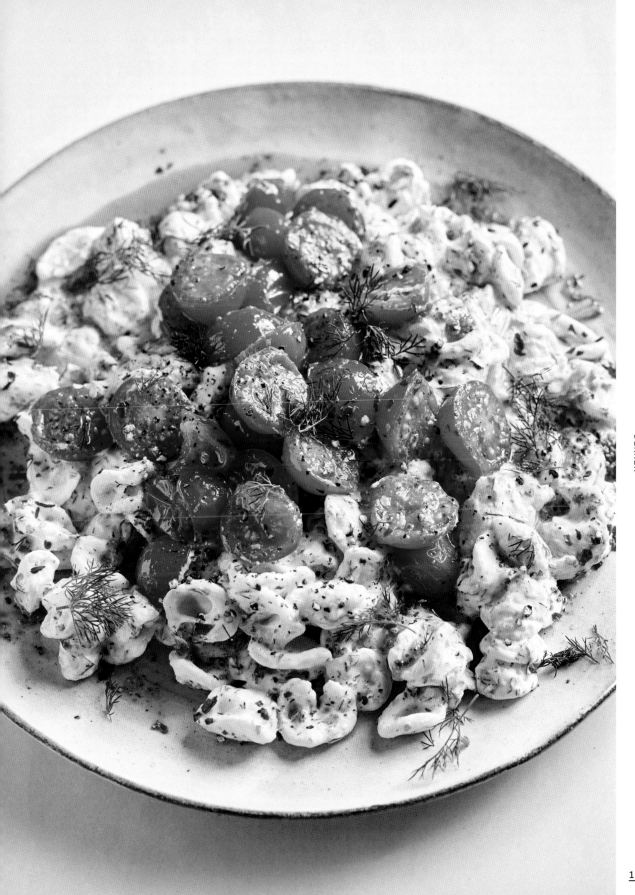

Good Gut Tacos

MAKES 12

Plant Diversity
Score: 6.75

Fish fingers are the star in this moreish midweek dish. The healthy fats in avocado and the fibre in the black beans and salad make this a wonderful gut-friendly dish. You can customise the salad vegetables according to your own or your children's preferences. If you don't have black beans, use a tin of kidney beans instead.

—

12 frozen jumbo fish fingers

Juice of 1 lime

1 small red onion, thinly sliced

12 cherry tomatoes, halved

1 ripe avocado, stoned and cut into small chunks

25g (1oz) coriander, finely chopped

1 x 400g (14oz) tin black beans, drained

½ tsp smoked paprika

1 tbsp olive oil

4 tbsp full-fat live Greek yoghurt or soured cream

60g (2½oz) pickled jalapeños, roughly chopped

12 crunchy taco shells or small corn and wheat tortilla wraps

1 little gem lettuce, shredded

Salt, to taste

1. Preheat the oven to 180°C fan/200°C/gas mark 6. Arrange the fish fingers on a baking tray and bake in the oven according to the packet instructions.

2. Rub the lime juice into the onion in a bowl and then add the tomatoes and avocado. Season with salt to taste. Scatter over half the coriander and keep this salad aside.

3. Refresh the beans by placing them in a sieve and pouring over some kettle-hot water. Tip the beans into a bowl and add the paprika, olive oil and salt to taste. Smash the beans slightly with the back of your fork to break them down a little.

4. Mix the yoghurt, jalapeños and remaining coriander together in a small bowl with a pinch of salt.

5. To assemble the tacos, start by placing a little shredded lettuce at the base of a crisp taco shell or tortilla wrap. Top with a fish finger, the smashed black beans, avocado salad and finally a drizzle of the jalapeño yoghurt.

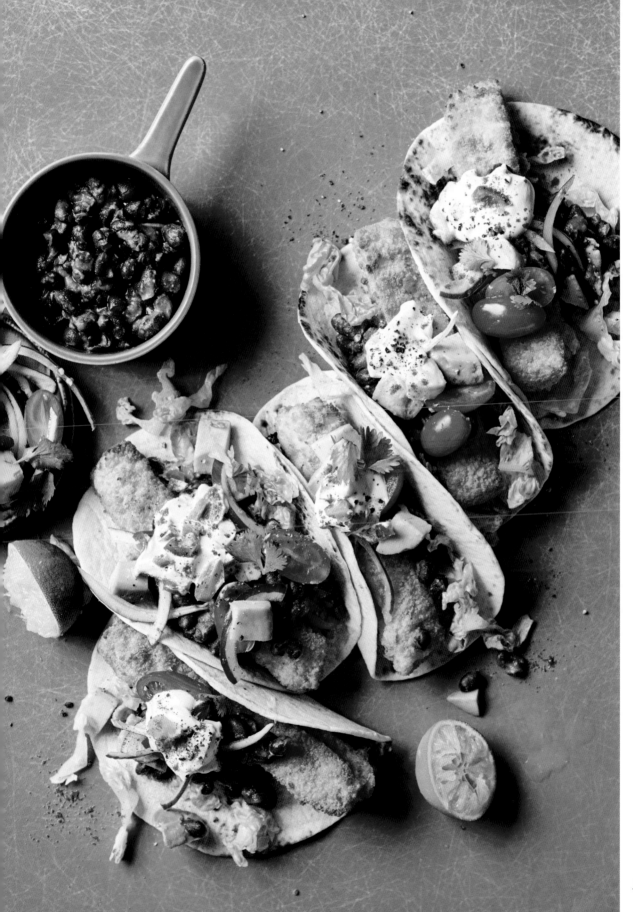

Levantine Aubergine + Chickpea Fatteh

SERVES 4

Plant Diversity
Score: 7
Bonus Score: 2.25

Fatteh is an Egyptian and Levantine sharing dish that consists of crispy bread chips topped with other ingredients, which vary by region. Think of them as dinner nachos from the Middle East – extremely moreish and full of textural contrasts. To make this as gut-healthy as possible, I have used wholewheat pitta instead of white and chickpeas and aubergine instead of fried chunks of lamb or beef mince. Baking the aubergines in a hot oven rather than frying means you avoid the addition of extra fat. Tahini and olive oil are both good sources of monounsaturated and polyunsaturated fats, which lower cholesterol and support heart health.

—

FOR THE PITTA CHIPS

4 wholewheat pitta breads cut into 4cm (1½in) squares

2 tbsp olive oil

½ tsp nigella seeds

FOR THE AUBERGINE

1 aubergine

2 tbsp olive oil

Salt, to taste

FOR THE CHICKPEAS

1 tbsp olive oil

1 white onion, thinly sliced

1 tsp garlic paste

1 tsp red chilli paste

1 x 400g (14oz) tin cherry tomatoes

1 x 400g (14oz) tin chickpeas, drained

1 tbsp tamarind paste

Pinch of sugar

FOR THE YOGHURT

200g (7oz) Greek yoghurt (or plant-based yoghurt)

2 heaped tbsp tahini

Juice of ½ lemon

TO SERVE

Handful of finely chopped parsley

Handful of pomegranate seeds

75g (2¾oz) toasted pine nuts

1. Preheat the oven to 180°C fan/200°C/gas mark 6. Put the pitta pieces into a bowl, drizzle with the olive oil and sprinkle over the nigella seeds, mixing well to ensure some oil has touched each piece of pitta bread. Scatter the pitta bread on to a baking tray and transfer to the oven to bake for 10–12 minutes, or until deep golden but not burnt. Remove from the oven and allow to cool slightly.

2. Meanwhile, cut the aubergine into bite-sized chunks (leave the skin on). Sprinkle with a little salt and drizzle over the olive oil, ensuring all the aubergine chunks are coated evenly. Transfer the aubergines to a baking tray and roast for 20 minutes until cooked through and golden at the edges.

3. Now for the chickpeas: heat the olive oil in a small saucepan over a medium heat and add the onion. After 10 minutes, when the onion has softened and become golden, add the garlic and chilli pastes and the cherry tomatoes. Stir well to combine and simmer for a few minutes before adding the chickpeas, about 200ml (7fl oz/generous ¾ cup) of kettle-hot water, the tamarind paste and a pinch of sugar. Braise for about 20 minutes until the mixture is thick, glossy and saucy. Season with salt to taste.

4. Combine the yoghurt with tahini, lemon juice and a touch of salt; stir well to make sure there are no lumps of tahini left. Loosen the mixture with a few tablespoons of kettle-hot water.

5. Assemble the dish on a large platter. Start at the base with the pitta chips, followed by the chickpeas and then a layer of the roasted aubergines. Spoon over the tahini yoghurt and dress with parsley, pomegranate seeds and toasted pine nuts.

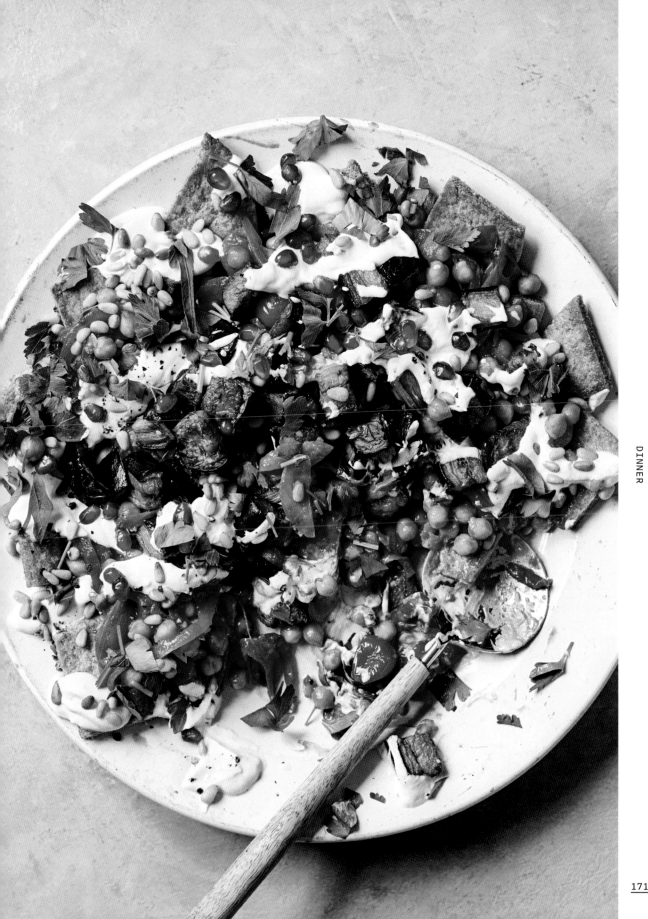

Sticky Jackfruit Burgers

SERVES 2

Plant Diversity
Score: 4.75

Burgers are a weakness of mine. They are, by their very design, made to be convenient and addictive, capturing our taste buds' attention effortlessly. This burger contains no cheese, no beef and no tomatoes, but don't be put off; it is packed with four different types of plants and a variety of delicious, sticky-sweet Korean inspired flavours. Jackfruit is a tropical fruit that is a wonderful vegan meat alternative; when unripe it has a firm texture and acts as a blank canvas for other flavours.

—

1 tsp garlic paste

1 tsp ginger paste

1 heaped tsp soft dark brown sugar

1 heaped tbsp gochujang paste

1 tbsp dark soy sauce

2 tsp apple cider vinegar (or rice vinegar)

½–1 tsp chilli flakes

100ml (3½fl oz/scant ½ cup) kettle-hot water

1 x 400g (14oz) tin green jackfruit, drained

1 tbsp vegetable oil

2 tbsp mayonnaise (or vegan mayo)

2 sesame-topped brioche buns

Salt, to taste

FOR THE SLAW

½ carrot, grated

¼ red cabbage, thinly sliced

6 mangetout, thinly sliced

1 tsp apple cider vinegar

1. Start by combining the garlic paste, ginger paste, sugar, gochujang paste, soy sauce, vinegar and chilli flakes in a saucepan with the water. Stir well and simmer for 5 minutes, or until it is bubbling, thick and sticky; it will thicken even more as it cool. Keep this gochujang sauce aside.

2. Dry the jackfruit on some strong kitchen paper. Drizzle the vegetable oil into a non-stick pan set over a high heat. Add the jackfruit to the oil and fry it on both sides for a few minutes, allowing it to take on some colour. When the jackfruit looks golden all over, add two-thirds of the prepared sauce and try to tease apart some of the jackfruit with a fork, so it has an almost 'pulled' appearance. After a minute or two, when the mixture looks rich and sticky, remove it from the heat. Taste and season with salt if needed.

3. Combine the carrot, cabbage and mangetout in a small bowl. Add the vinegar and season with salt to taste. Combine the remaining gochujang sauce with the mayonnaise. Toast the brioche buns.

4. To assemble the burgers, start with the pulled jackfruit at the base. Top with the slaw and then the gochujang mayo. Place the burger lid on top and you are ready to eat the most exciting plant-based, gut-loving burger of your life!

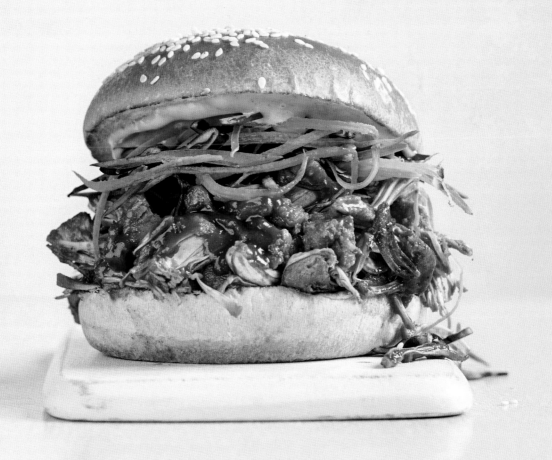

Shawarma Pan Chicken with Lentil + Pickled Vegetable Salad

Plant Diversity
Score: 7.5

Say goodbye to your Friday night chicken doner on the way home, and say hello to this vibrant, gut-friendly dish inspired by chicken shawarma. All the flavours of a doner kebab are there, thanks to the shawarma seasoning, but the accompaniment of lentils, prebiotic red cabbage and pickled vegetables makes this dish a treat, not just for your taste buds, but also for your gut.

—

FOR THE CHICKEN

1 tsp coriander seeds

1 tsp dried oregano

½ tsp grated nutmeg

1 tsp garlic granules

1 tsp chilli flakes

½ tsp ground cardamom

½ tsp ground cinnamon

10 grinds of black pepper

800g–1kg (1lb 12oz–2lb 4oz) chicken thigh fillets, skin removed

2 tbsp olive oil

Salt, to taste

FOR THE LENTILS

250g (9oz) red cabbage, finely shredded

200g (7oz) jarred mixed vegetable pickles (turnips, carrots, cucumbers, cauliflower etc.)

500g (1lb 2oz) cooked Puy lentils (from a pouch or tin)

1 tbsp olive oil

Handful of finely chopped parsley leaves

FOR THE CHILLI SAUCE

300g (10oz) roasted red peppers from a jar

1 tbsp rose harissa paste

1 tbsp olive oil

Toasted pitta breads, to serve (optional)

1. Combine the coriander seeds, oregano, nutmeg, garlic granules, chilli flakes, cardamom, cinnamon and black pepper in a pestle and mortar and give the mixture a good grind to break the coriander seeds down. Dust the chicken thighs all over with the spice mix, ensuring the chicken is coated evenly. If any of the chicken is thicker than about 2.5cm (1in), give it a good bash with a rolling pin to thin it down.

2. Heat a non-stick frying pan over a medium-high heat. Add the olive oil, followed by the spice-coated chicken (you may need to add the chicken in batches as you are looking for a really deep golden crust to form on the surface, to add flavour and texture). Season the chicken with salt to taste. Fry the chicken for about 8 minutes on each side, then remove the pan from the heat and allow the chicken to rest for a short time before slicing into small chunks.

3. Add the red cabbage to a bowl and season it with salt. Take a few tablespoons of the liquid from the pickled vegetables jar and, with your hands, give the cabbage a good scrunch, so as to release the purple pigments and soften it down a little.

4. Heat the lentils in the microwave or with a few splashes of water in a saucepan on the hob. Drop the lentils into the bowl of cabbage and drizzle over the olive oil. Mix well and top with the pickled vegetables from the jar and the chopped parsley.

5. Blend the roasted peppers, harissa paste and olive oil with a touch of salt to form a smooth, spicy pepper sauce.

6. Serve the chicken with the warm lentil and veg salad and the spicy sauce. Pitta bread on the side is an option if you feel the dish needs it, although I must admit I don't miss the pitta bread if it is not there. You can eat any leftover chicken in lettuce cups for lunch the next day.

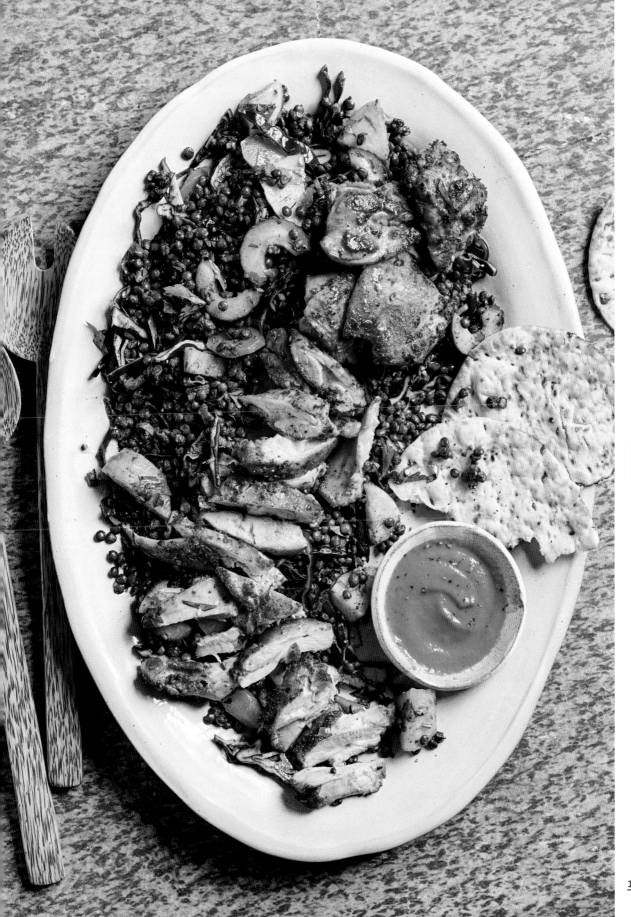

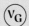

Creamy Cashew + Sun-dried Tomato Pasta with Dukkah

SERVES 4

Plant Diversity
Score: 4.75

This dish really hits the spot: intensely creamy (despite not actually using cream) and with a deep umami flavour from the sun-dried tomatoes and nutritional yeast flakes, a useful vegan ingredient that lends a nutty, cheesy flavour to dishes. Dukkah is a fragrant, roasted Egyptian spice and nut blend, adding textural crunch to an already spectacular dish. I use wholewheat penne here but feel free to use any pasta of your choice. For extra plant diversity, you can serve this dish with a fresh cherry tomato and rocket salad on the side. It eats very well cold the next day too.

—

300g (10oz) wholewheat penne

100g (3½oz) cashews

200g (7oz) sun-dried tomatoes, drained from their oil

3 garlic cloves

1 heaped tsp hot paprika (or ½ tsp chilli flakes)

2 tbsp nutritional yeast (or vegetarian hard-style Italian cheese)

1 tsp dried oregano

4 heaped tsp dukkah (see Note)

Salt, to taste

1. Start by bringing a large saucepan of water to the boil. When the water is boiling, add a generous sprinkling of salt. Add the penne and cook until al dente (or follow the packet instructions). Drain, reserving the pasta water.

2. Combine the cashews, sun-dried tomatoes, garlic, paprika, nutritional yeast and oregano together in a blender. Add about 4 ladles of pasta water and blend to form a creamy, smooth sauce. Season with salt to taste.

3. Pour the cashew and sun-dried tomato sauce into the pan you used to boil the pasta. Simmer it gently for about 4 minutes to allow all the flavours to develop further. If it looks too thick, do not hesitate to add a little more of the reserved pasta water. Tumble the pasta into the sauce and stir well to combine. Serve with dukkah sprinkled over the top.

NOTE

You'll find ready-made dukkah in most large supermarkets but if you feel like making your own , coarsely blend 75g (2¾oz) toasted hazelnuts with 2 tablespoons of toasted sesame seeds, 1 tablespoon of toasted cumin seeds, 1 teaspoon of toasted fennel seeds, ½ teaspoon of toasted black peppercorns and 1 heaped teaspoon of coriander seeds.

the kitchen prescription

Cashew nuts (Anacardium occidentale L.)

+ Cashews are rich in copper, an element which is vital for bone health and the creation of collagen (the connective tissue that makes the scaffolding for bones). It is also thought to benefit our memory and brain function.

+ Although more studies are needed, it seems as though cashews may beneficially impact cholesterol levels in the blood and are therefore considered a heart-healthy food item.

Crispy Gnocchi with Creamy Turmeric + Spinach Sauce

SERVES 2

```
Plant Diversity
Score: 3
Bonus Score: 1
```

There is something deeply satisfying about crunchy, golden, crispy fried gnocchi cascading into a pillowy cloud of turmeric-hued golden sauce. I sometimes make this dish when I am unwell and feel like I need the extra carbohydrates for energy and the anti-inflammatory properties of turmeric to lift my spirits and health. The addition of black pepper is intentional; its presence makes the turmeric more bioavailable (meaning the proportion of the healthy compounds in the turmeric that can enter our circulation is increased), not to mention that they taste great together. For more detail on dietary carbohydrates, see page 15.

—

50g (2oz) butter

500g (1lb 2oz) ready-made gnocchi

1 tbsp olive oil

½ white onion, finely chopped

1 garlic clove, finely chopped

80g (3oz) baby spinach

175ml (6fl oz/¾ cup) double cream

½ tsp ground turmeric (or a small piece of grated fresh turmeric)

50g (2oz/½ cup) grated Parmesan (or vegetarian hard-style Italian cheese)

½ tsp coarse black pepper

1 tbsp toasted sunflower seeds (optional)

1. Melt the butter in a frying pan; when the butter starts bubbling, add the gnocchi. Allow the gnocchi and cook until golden on all sides, this takes about 5–7 minutes. Remove the gnocchi from the pan and set aside.

2. Add the olive oil the same pan, followed by the onion and garlic. Fry the onion for 5 minutes over a low heat until it is a light golden brown. Now add the spinach leaves and allow them to wilt. Pour the cream into the wilted spinach, followed by the turmeric, Parmesan and black pepper. Stir well to combine and when the cream has just heated through, take the sauce off the heat. Tumble in the gnocchi and scatter over the sunflower seeds (if using).

DINNER

Tandoori Chicken Traybake

SERVES 4

Plant Diversity
Score: 8

Dependable deliciousness – this is a recipe I turn to time and time again. If you don't have the ingredients to make your own tandoori marinade, by all means buy one instead. Feel free to use any vegetables of your choice to customise this.

—

2 red onions, chopped into thick chunks

1 leek, chopped into 2.5cm (1in) rings

2 carrots, peeled and chopped into 3cm (1¼in) chunks

2 peppers (any colour), deseeded and quartered

1kg (2lb 4oz) chicken thighs

1 x 400g (14oz) tin chickpeas, drained (optional)

Salt, to taste

FOR THE TANDOORI MARINADE

1 heaped tsp mild chilli powder

1 heaped tsp mild paprika

1 tsp tomato purée

2 tsp garlic paste

1 tsp ginger paste

1 heaped tsp cumin seeds

1 tsp garam masala

Juice of 1 lemon

4 generous tbsp extra-virgin olive oil

FOR THE CUCUMBER RAITA

1 small cucumber, grated

400g (14oz) live natural yoghurt

1 tsp cumin seeds

1. Preheat the oven to 180°C fan/200°C/gas mark 6. Combine all the ingredients for the marinade in a small bowl, stir well and set aside.

2. Tumble the onions, leek, carrots and peppers on to the base of a large roasting tray. Drizzle half the marinade over the vegetables and mix well to ensure that all the vegetables are coated evenly.

3. Place the chicken thighs in the bowl with the remaining marinade and turn to coat evenly in the marinade. Lay the chicken over the vegetables and sprinkle with salt to taste. Cover the roasting try with foil and bake in the oven for 35 minutes.

4. Take the chicken out of the oven and remove the foil. Toss in the chickpeas (if using) and baste the chicken with the pan juices. Increase the oven temperature to 200°C fan/220°C/gas mark 7 and return the roasting tray to the oven for a further 25 minutes, or until the vegetables are charred and jammy.

5. Meanwhile, squeeze the moisture out of the grated cucumber and then combine it with the yoghurt and cumin seeds in a bowl. Season with salt to taste and serve alongside the traybake.

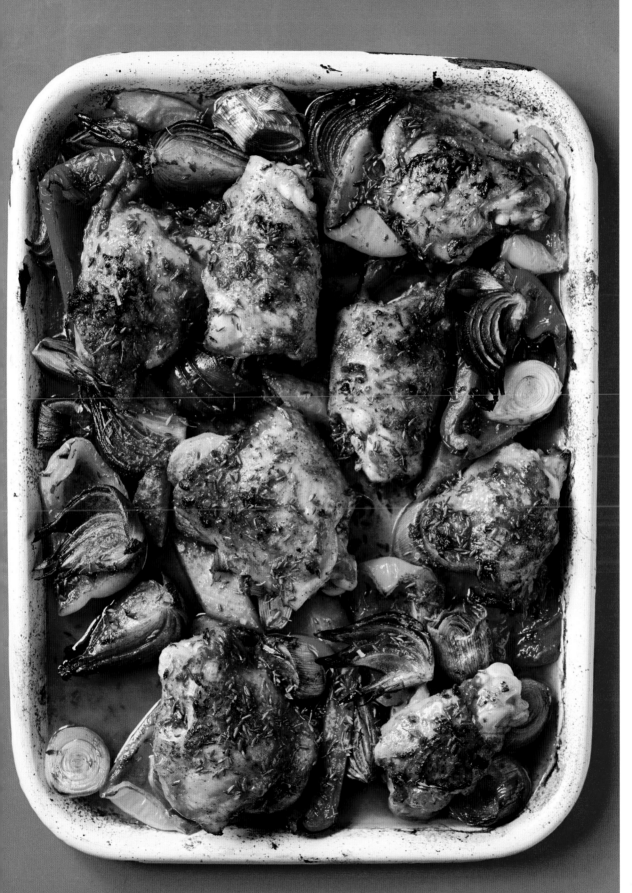

Broccoli Spaghetti with Herby Chermoula

SERVES 4

Plant Diversity
Score: 7.5

Chermoula is a versatile North African relish, usually used to flavour fish or meat. Most people will not have tried it with pasta but it works almost like a North African-inspired pesto and provides a welcome change of flavours to the usual ones that we associate with spaghetti. I've added nuts and seeds to the chermoula in order to enrich it with gut-loving fibre – plus I've used wholewheat spaghetti.

—

250g (9oz) wholewheat spaghetti

300g (10oz) broccoli, cut into small florets

Salt, to taste

FOR THE OLIVE, SEED AND PISTACHIO CHERMOULA

75g (2¾oz) coriander

75g (2¾oz) parsley

75g (2¾oz) pitted green olives

1–2 small preserved lemons

3 garlic cloves

1 tsp chilli flakes

2 tbsp toasted mixed seeds

2 tsp cumin seeds

3 tbsp shelled pistachios (or pine nuts)

8–10 tbsp extra-virgin olive oil

FOR THE TOPPING

75g (2¾oz) crumbled feta cheese

Handful of sun-dried tomatoes, finely diced

BONUS GUT-FRIENDLY ADDITIONS

Instead of broccoli, use whichever vegetables you have to hand: sauté some cherry tomatoes, peppers, spinach or mushrooms before adding the chermoula.

1. Cook the spaghetti in a large saucepan of salted boiling water according to the packet instructions. About 2–3 minutes before the spaghetti is done, add the broccoli to the boiling pasta water. Drain the spaghetti and broccoli, reserving a cup or so of the pasta water.

2. Put all the ingredients for the chermoula, except the olive oil, into a food processor. Blitz until all the ingredients have combined well and no large coarse bits remain. Now pour in the olive oil and pulse briefly to combine.

3. Add two-thirds of the chermoula to the same pan that you cooked the pasta in and place over a medium heat. When it starts bubbling, add the spaghetti and broccoli and toss well. To loosen the mixture, add some of the reserved pasta water, then season with salt to taste. Serve immediately, topped with crumbled feta cheese and sun-dried tomatoes.

NOTE
Keep the remaining chermoula in the fridge and use as a topping for baked sweet potatoes (page 148).

Olives

+ Olives are rich in polyphenols like oleocanthal, which has antioxidant properties and may behave like a natural anti-inflammatory.

+ Fatty acids like oleic acid found in olives are also thought to reduce the risk of heart disease, reduce blood pressure, and help regulate cholesterol.

+ It is easy to overlook the fact that olives are in fact a popular fermented food item, rich in Lactobacillus, a type of gut-friendly bacteria.

+ I would advise eating moderate amounts of olives as the curing/brining process does introduce a fair amount of salt.

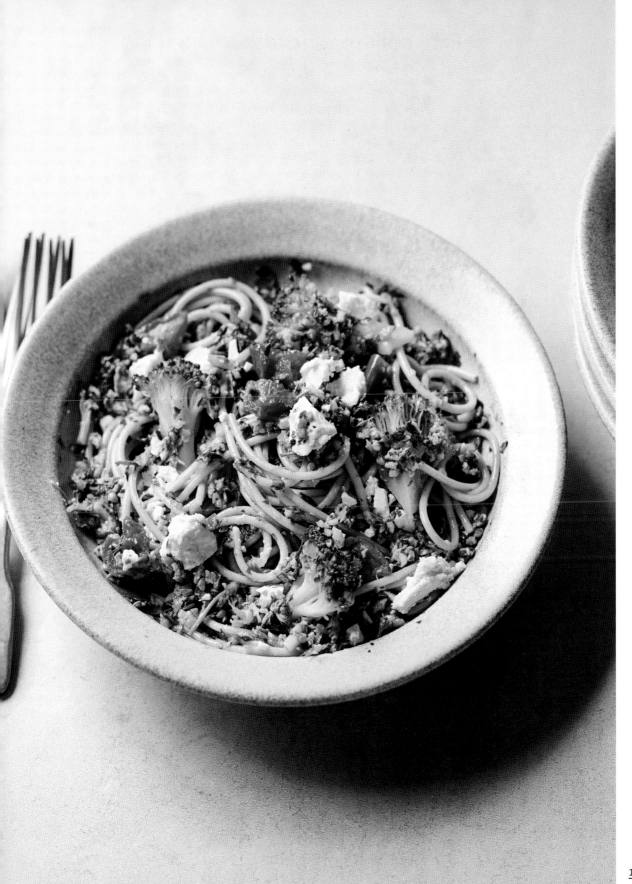

Gut-healing Masala Cottage Pie

SERVES 4
(WITH LEFTOVERS)

Plant Diversity
Score: 14.75

Who can deny the comfort of a good cottage pie? The creamy mash hides the umami-rich interior, and the combination of both is one of the best things to come out of British cuisine. Really perfect for a weekend dinner. This gut-loving version has the added advantage of contributing to your gut health; the vast range of vegetables and legumes used, along with the addition of anti-inflammatory turmeric make it a terrific gut-healthy alternative to conventional cottage pie. To maximise the fibre content, I have intentionally left half the potato skins on.

—

3 tbsp extra-virgin olive oil

1 onion, finely chopped

3 garlic cloves, crushed

1 leek, finely diced

1 celery stick, finely diced

1 red pepper, finely diced

½ carrot, finely diced

½ tsp ground turmeric

1 tsp toasted cumin seeds

1 tsp mild–medium chilli powder

1 tsp garam masala

½ tsp dried oregano

1 x 400g (14oz) tin cherry tomatoes

1 vegetable stock cube

100g (3½oz/½ cup) dried green lentils

50g (2oz/¼ cup) brown lentils

50g (2oz/¼ cup) red lentils

1 x 400g (14oz) tin pinto beans, drained

Salt, to taste

FOR THE MASH

800g (1lb 12oz) Maris Piper potatoes

1 tsp ground turmeric

25g (1oz) finely chopped coriander

1 tsp cumin seeds

50g (2oz) butter

125ml (4fl oz/½ cup) warm milk

50g (2oz/½ cup) grated mature Cheddar cheese

1. Preheat the oven to 180°C fan/200°C/gas mark 6.

2. Heat the olive oil in a saucepan over a medium heat. Add the onion and garlic and sauté for 5 minutes until the onion has softened and started to take on some colour. Now add the leek, celery, red pepper and carrot and stir well. Sweat the vegetables for about 7 minutes until they are soft and jammy.

3. At this point, add the turmeric, cumin seeds, chilli powder, garam masala and oregano. This will transform the vegetables completely. Add the tinned cherry tomatoes to the vegetables along with the stock cube and 600ml (20fl oz/2½ cups) of kettle-hot water. When the mixture has come to the boil, add the three types of dried lentils. Stir well and simmer for about 20 minutes, or until the lentils have cooked through (if they still haven't lost their bite after 20 minutes, continue to cook for another 5–10 minutes). If the mixture starts looking too dry at any point, add a touch more water; you are aiming for a thick, gravy-like consistency. To complete the dish, add the drained pinto beans, season with salt to taste and spoon the mixture into a pie dish.

4. Peel half the potatoes and leave the skin on for the other half. Chop them into even-sized chunks and boil them in a saucepan for about 12 minutes, or until they are cooked through. Drain in a colander and return the potatoes to the pan. Add the turmeric, coriander, cumin seeds, butter and milk to the potatoes and season with salt to taste. Mash the potatoes until everything is well combined, then spoon the potatoes over the lentil mixture and sprinkle over the cheese. Transfer to the oven for 30 minutes, or until the surface is brown and crunchy in places.

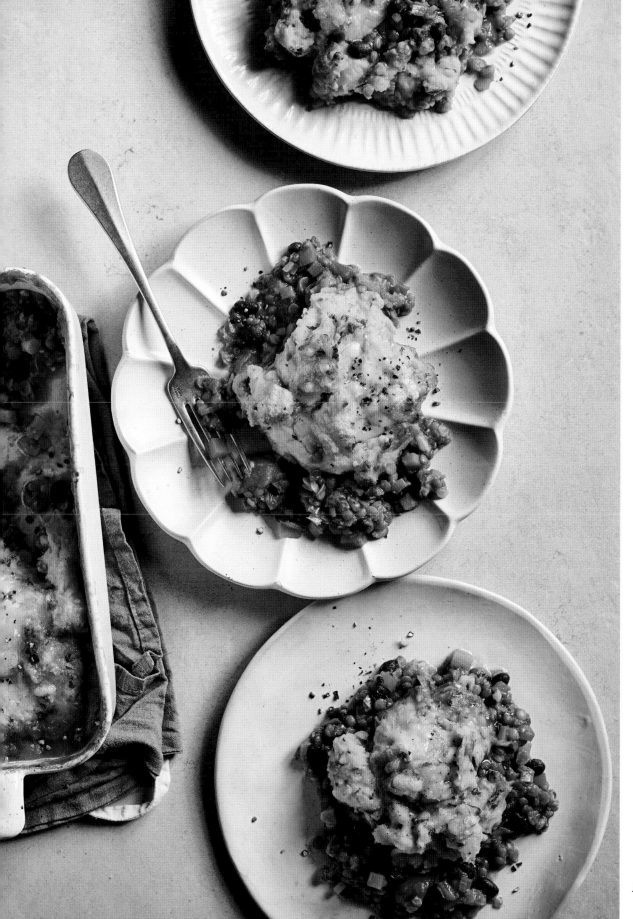

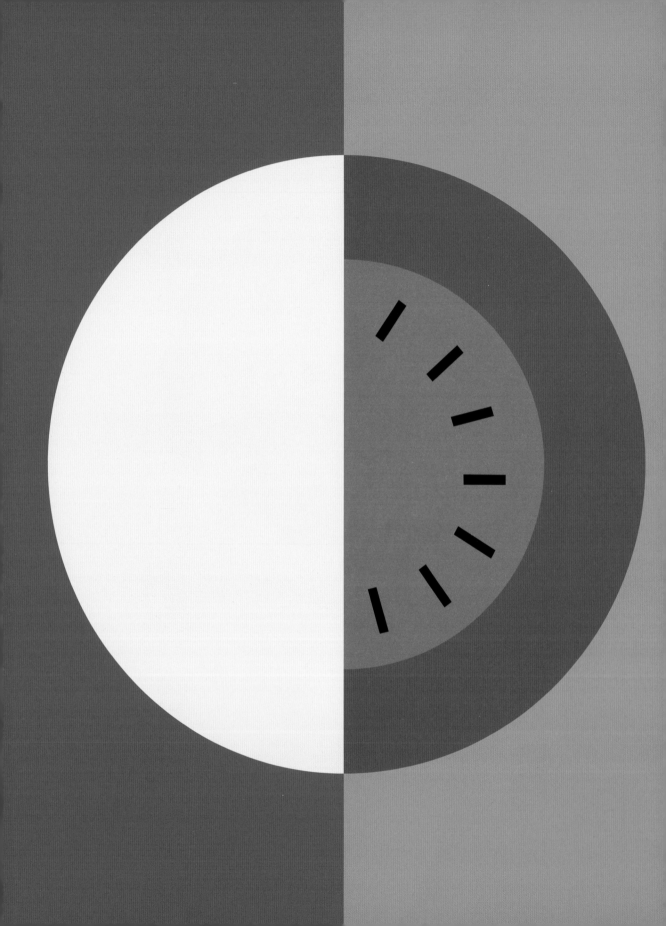

MEZZE

Sharing* platters to boost gut microbial diversity

Eating is all about community. Almost every society on earth has woven a sharing element into the fabric of their culinary culture, and none is more focused on commensality, the act of eating together, than mezze.

Mezze (or mezzeh, or mazzah) is a casual, unpretentious style of dining not dissimilar to Spanish tapas, which is found in all the cuisines of the former Ottoman Empire. The dishes are usually cold to start, often vegetarian, and served with chunks of hot, fresh bread. A bite of mezze can transport you to anywhere within a thousand miles of Constantinople; hummus from Egypt, tabbouleh from the Levant, dolma from Crete – the list goes on.

It's no accident that mezze is as gut-friendly a form of dining as it gets; an array of plant-based dishes next to probiotic dairy products like labneh alongside leguminous dips like hummus are naturally fibre-dense, wholesome and bound to be great for your gut. The numerous small plates served are lively, designed to stimulate the appetite, keep the taste buds guessing as well as celebrating plant-rather than diversity in the diet. Soul-searching, intimate conversations and raucous laughter envelop eaters from every corner of a dinner table, covered with food of every colour under the sun.

My three key pointers to setting up a gut-friendly mezze evening at home would be:

1.	Choose at least three or four key mezze items for the night. Consider serving them on a large platter, rather than separate small dishes so that people can share from the same plate. They take next to no time to prepare, which is always a bonus.
2.	Include an array of rainbow-coloured vegetables with your mezze, like Persian cucumbers, radishes, mooli, ripe tomatoes and olives in order to optimise gut microbial diversity for you and your guests.
3.	You can never have enough warm bread at a mezze night. Keep the home -made flatbreads, pitta or lavash breads coming, and serve them with some good-quality peppery olive oil.

Mezze is a tactile, sensorial experience that allows you to slow right down, savour each mouthful and linger for as long as you wish. A mezze platter encourages the practice of mindful eating – an approach to eating which focuses on sensory awareness and the experience of eating, on savouring what is in your mouth, and encouraging your full mental presence in that moment, acknowledging the tastes and textures that you are experiencing. I believe that a mindful approach to eating can help you foster good gut health; there is evidence that those who practise this approach often eat less, relish the food they are eating, and select foods which have more desirable health benefits. The success of mindful eating is not measured in kilos lost; instead, success is found by engaging fully in the process of eating itself.

Here is a simple mindful exercise that you can practise with any of the mezze dishes in this chapter.

+ Imagine you have just been dropped off on this planet, and you know nothing about where you are. You have never experienced anything from Earth, it is all new to you. Take a few deep breaths and relax.
+ Look at the bread and pick it up. Feel its weight and examine its surface – the various toasted parts, doughy centre, its crumbs; really look at this object, as if it is the first time you are looking at it.
+ Smell this object and notice how you react. Squeeze the bread between your fingers and see if you can hear what sound it makes. Notice what you are feeling about this object.
+ Looking carefully, dip the bread into the mezze and slowly bring it to your mouth. Just hold it there for a few moments. What do you notice?
Let the mezze roll into your mouth, but do not chew yet. Allow yourself to taste the mezze and bread. Notice your salivation and how your body is responding.
+ Now bite down, just once. What do you notice?
+ Slowly begin to chew, noticing what each bite brings. Chew the mezze and bread slowly and deliberately, then swallow. Close your eyes for a few moments to understand the significance of what you just experienced.

Fresh Persian Herb Platter

SERVES 4-6

Plant Diversity
Score: 6
Bonus Score: 0.25

This herb platter, known as *sabzi khordan* is served at most Persian meals as an appetiser, often taking the place of a salad. It is essentially made up of a selection of fresh herbs, radishes, spring onions and cheese. Served with a flatbread called lavash, it is probably one of, if not the boldest and most punchy flavoured of all sharing platters. I have made a few tweaks to the classic recipe, making it even more gut friendly than before. Overall this recipe has a very pleasing effort-to-reward ratio; the most laborious part is washing the herbs.

I've suggested herbs to use below but you can chop and change these according to preference and availability; just aim for at least three different herbs.

—

Large bunch of fresh parsley

Small bunch of tarragon leaves

Small bunch of basil leaves

Small bunch of mint

Small bunch of sorrel leaves (if available)

200g (7oz) block of feta cheese

250g (9oz) jarred balls of labneh in olive oil

1 heaped tbsp za'atar

3 tbsp extra-virgin olive oil

10 radishes

6 spring onions, roots trimmed and cut in half crossways

250g (9oz) walnuts, soaked in water for 5 hours (or overnight), then drained

1 cucumber, sliced into 1cm (½in) thick rounds

Warmed lavash bread or pitta bread, to serve

1. Rinse your herbs, if necessary, and pat dry.

2. Place the feta, labneh, za'atar and olive oil in separate small serving dishes. Place these serving dishes on a large platter.

3. Arrange the herbs, radishes, spring onions, walnuts and cucumber artfully around the dishes. Serve with the lavash or pitta bread.

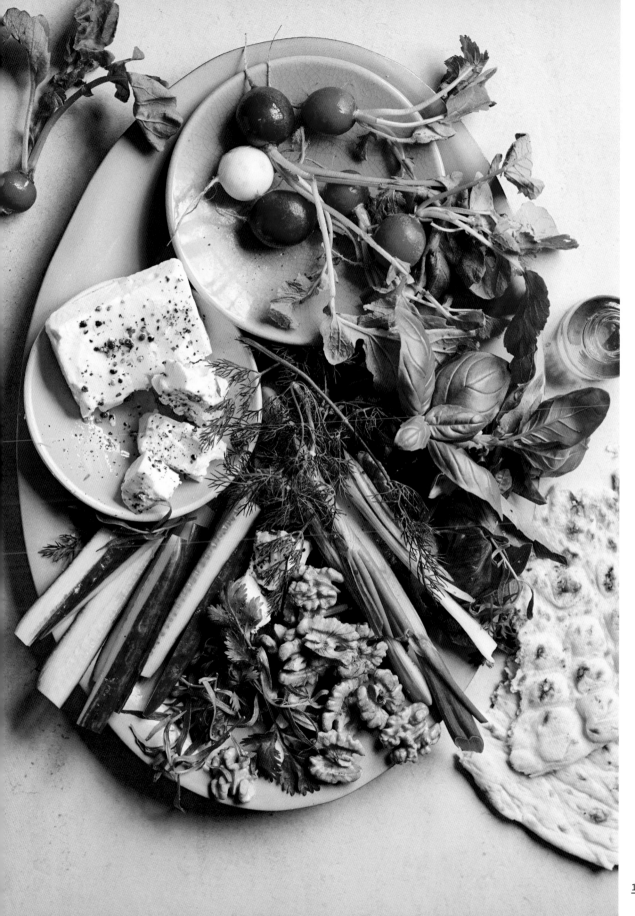

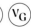

Charred Courgettes with Garlic Yoghurt

SERVES 4-6

Plant Diversity
Score: 1.75
Bonus Score: 2

3 tbsp extra-virgin olive oil

3 courgettes, sliced into 1.5cm (⅝in) thick rounds

1 level tsp white sugar

1 tsp coarse black pepper

1 whole small garlic bulb

250g (9oz) full-fat live Greek yoghurt (or plant-based yoghurt)

Salt, to taste

1 tsp dried rose petals, to garnish (optional)

BONUS GUT-FRIENDLY TOPPINGS

40g (1½oz) golden sultanas, soaked in warm water

40g (1½oz) shelled pistachios, roughly chopped

Here intense heat caramelises the sugars in the courgettes until they blister and char, heightening their complex bitter tones. You can also make this with peppers, carrots or aubergines if you prefer and if you are vegan, substitute a good-quality coconut yoghurt instead of the Greek yoghurt. Toasted pine nuts or almonds will also work if pistachios are not available (or too pricey). Serve with toasted pitta bread or any other flatbread of your choice. In summer use a barbecue instead of the oven.

—

1. Preheat the oven to 220°C fan/240°C/gas mark 8.

2. Drizzle 2 tablespoons of the olive oil as evenly as possible over the courgettes, then sprinkle over the sugar and season with salt and the pepper. Place the courgettes in a single layer on a large baking sheet lined with baking paper. (If you have small baking trays you may need two of them.) Slice off the top of the garlic bulb around 2cm (¾in) from its stem, and drizzle a tablespoon of olive oil into the cloves. Place the whole garlic on the baking tray alongside the courgettes. Transfer to the oven and bake for about 30 minutes, or until deeply charred. Remove from the oven and allow to cool.

3. Squeeze the baked garlic to release the cooked garlic pods from the papery skin – you don't have to use them all if you don't like your food too garlicky but I tend to use most of it. Mix the garlic into the yoghurt and then season with a touch of salt.

4. To serve, spread the yoghurt over a serving platter. Top with the charred courgettes and scatter over the golden sultanas, pistachios and rose petals (if using).

the kitchen prescription

Garlic (Allium sativum L.)

+ The medicinal properties of garlic are thought to be wielded by an active compound called allicin, a pungent, almost sulphurous smelling compound.

+ Garlic is thought to exert a positive impact on heart health; it reduces cholesterol, impacts the clumping of platelets that are involved in blood clotting, and may possess blood pressure-reducing

and cholesterol-lowering properties.

+ Different compounds in garlic are thought to promote human health through their anti-microbial and anti-tumour effects. Additionally, other compounds appear to be beneficial for blood sugar regulation. However, the exact mechanisms are not always understood, and more research is needed.

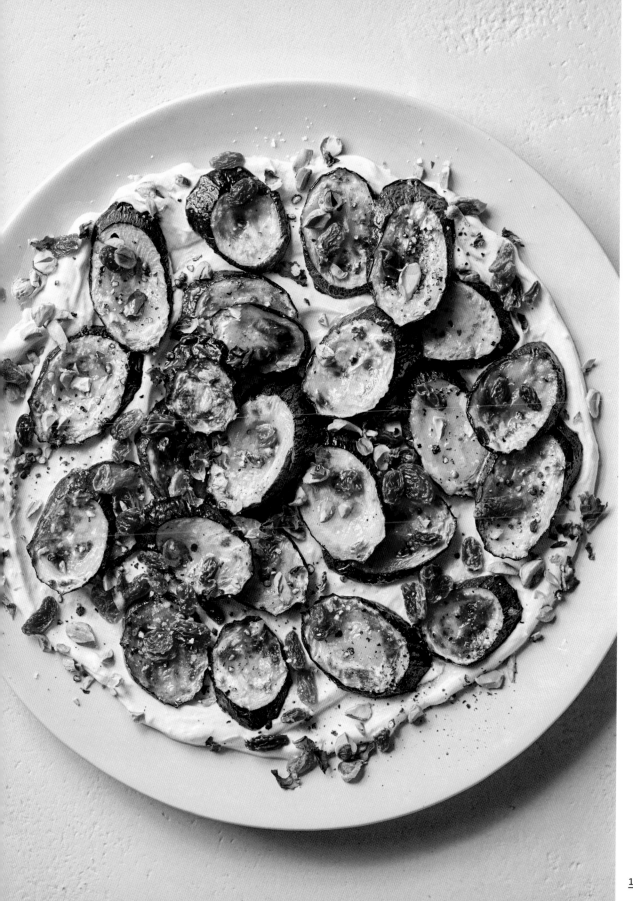

Fiery Red Pepper Mezze

SERVES 4–6

Plant Diversity
Score: 5.25
Bonus Score: 0.25

I originally made this recipe as a vegetable side dish for a chicken curry, but there was so much left over that most of it went straight into my fridge. The following day, I unexpectedly had some friends visit after work and these leftover peppers were all I had to hand. To my delight they tasted even better the next day, straight out of the fridge and spread on to a mezze platter.

—

3 tbsp olive oil

200g (7oz) white onion, thinly sliced

½ tsp ground turmeric

1 tsp cumin seeds

½ tsp fennel seeds (optional)

½ tsp medium red chilli powder

150g (5oz) cherry tomatoes, halved

3 peppers (ideally red and yellow), thinly sliced

1 tsp amchoor (mango powder) or the juice of ½ lemon

1 tsp maple syrup, to taste

Salt, to taste

1. Heat the olive oil in a saucepan, add the onion and fry over a medium heat for 6–8 minutes, or until it starts turning a deep golden colour. Add the turmeric, cumin seeds, fennel seeds (if using) and chilli powder and stir well, ensuring the spices don't stick to the pan. If it looks like they are about to catch, add a few tablespoons of warm water.

2. Next, add the cherry tomatoes and cook down for a further 10 minutes until the tomatoes have broken down and the oil has split out to form a sort of 'masala'. You will need to keep stirring the mixture at this stage.

3. Now add the peppers and cook for 12 minutes to allow the peppers to soften. Add 100ml (3½fl oz/scant ½ cup) warm water and braise for a further 10 minutes until the peppers have a soft, jammy consistency. To complete the dish, season with salt to taste, the amchoor (mango powder) or lemon juice for tartness and a touch of maple syrup, if needed, for rounded sweetness.

the kitchen prescription

Peppers (Capsicum annuum)

+ Not all peppers are created equal; nutritional content will vary according to their colour. For example, immature green peppers are felt to be more polyphenol-rich than mature red peppers, while red peppers are felt to be richer in potassium, folate and vitamin C than yellow or green varieties.

+ There are some studies suggesting that carotenoids found in peppers called lutein and zeaxanthin can help your vision by preventing cataracts forming and the macula at the back of the eye from degenerating.

+ Early evidence in human-focused studies seems to be pointing to red peppers having a beneficial effect on reducing metabolic syndrome, a precursor to developing diabetes.

Turkish Carrots in Saffron Sauce

SERVES 4-6

Plant Diversity
Score: 2
Bonus Score: 1

While on holiday in Istanbul, I was lucky enough to be invited for a meal at a Turkish family's home. The experience opened my eyes to the tenderness with which the Turks treat their produce. In particular, vegetable dishes were prepared simply yet skilfully, often making them the centre point of the table. This dish would be equally confident sitting beside a plate of grilled meat, but it is as a mezze dish alongside warm, sesame encrusted bread where it truly shines.

—

2 tbsp olive oil, plus extra for drizzling

350g (12oz) grated carrots

300g (10oz) kefir yoghurt (or plant-based yoghurt)

1 fat garlic clove, grated

½ tsp maple syrup

½ tsp chilli flakes (use pul biber Turkish chilli flakes if you have them)

Pinch of saffron (ground, then steeped in a few tbsp of warm water for a few hours)

Salt, to taste

BONUS GUT-FRIENDLY TOPPINGS

Handful of toasted, roughly chopped hazelnuts or pistachio slivers

1. Place the olive oil and carrots in a saucepan and heat over a medium-high heat for about 3–5 minutes. You don't want to cook the carrots fully, rather, just to soften them slightly and release some of their aroma and trapped flavours. Take the carrots off the heat, transfer to a bowl and allow to cool.

2. Mix the kefir yoghurt, garlic, maple syrup, chilli flakes and saffron water into the carrots and season generously with salt. You can drizzle with a little extra olive oil and chopped nuts to garnish if desired.

MEZZE

the kitchen prescription

Saffron (Crocus sativus L.)

+ In Chinese medicine saffron has been used for its medicinal, aphrodisiac and anti-spasmodic effects for centuries.

+ Chemical analysis of the plant shows it is complex, with over 150 volatile and non-volatile compounds. The major bioactive compounds are safranal, crocin and picrocrocin, which give it that unique aroma and bitter taste.

+ Small studies have suggested that saffron may be helpful in relieving the symptoms of premenstrual syndrome if used over three to four cycles.

+ There is emerging evidence that saffron extracts might have some beneficial anti-depressant effects in mild to moderate depression states, however more research is needed before any formal recommendations can be made.

Sour + Sticky Tamarind Aubergines

SERVES 4–6

Plant Diversity
Score: 2
Bonus Score: 3

Aubergines are the berry of the Solanum melongena plant. Their culinary gift is the ability to absorb fat and flavour; to cook the most gut-healthy aubergines, therefore, bake them in a light coating of oil rather than shallow- or deep-frying them, as they will absorb huge amounts of oil in the latter. Try to use the aubergine skin as well as the flesh in your recipes. The skin is full of fibre and the purple pigment, anthocyanin, is thought to exert powerful antioxidant effects, which protect our tissues from damage. It is thought that cooking only slightly reduces the anthocyanins, so the more skin, the better.

—

2 medium aubergines, sliced into finger-shaped slices (like chips)

3 tbsp extra-virgin olive oil

1 tsp mild or medium chilli powder

1 tsp miso paste

4 tbsp tamarind paste or chutney (or use 2 tbsp pomegranate molasses)

3 tbsp maple syrup

1 tsp tomato purée

Salt, to taste

BONUS GUT-FRIENDLY TOPPINGS

1 spring onion, thinly sliced

1 tbsp toasted sesame seeds or roughly chopped peanuts

1 tbsp pomegranate seeds

1. Preheat the oven to 200°C fan/220°C/gas mark 7 and line a baking tray with baking paper.

2. Toss the aubergines with the olive oil and a pinch of salt and scatter over the lined tray in an even layer. Bake in the oven for 30 minutes until they have cooked through and taken on some colour.

3. While the aubergines are cooking, combine the chilli powder, miso paste, tamarind paste, maple syrup, tomato purée and 200ml (7fl oz/ generous ¾ cup) kettle-hot water in a bowl; stir well to combine. Transfer the mixture to a frying pan and boil for 4–5 minutes until a thick, sticky glaze forms.

4. Remove the aubergines from the oven and transfer them immediately to the bowl of sticky glaze. Toss everything together well to ensure all the aubergine is coated. Garnish with a scattering of sliced spring onion, toasted sesame seeds or peanuts and pomegranate seeds.

the kitchen prescription

Tamarind (Tamarindus indica)

+ The tamarind tree produces a brown pod-like fruit which has a tart, sweet pulp. It is used extensively in South Asian, South East Asian and Far Eastern cuisines to add flavour to curries, chutneys and more.

+ The antioxidant properties of tamarind are impressive; if animal studies are to be believed, tamarind may help reverse fatty liver disease.

+ Extracts of tamarind seeds are thought to help regulate blood sugar in diabetics.

+ Tamarind contains a compound called lupeol, which has shown some promise in animal studies as anti-inflammatory and anti-microbial.

+ In traditional medicine, tamarind has been used to treat malaria (though I wouldn't rely on it).

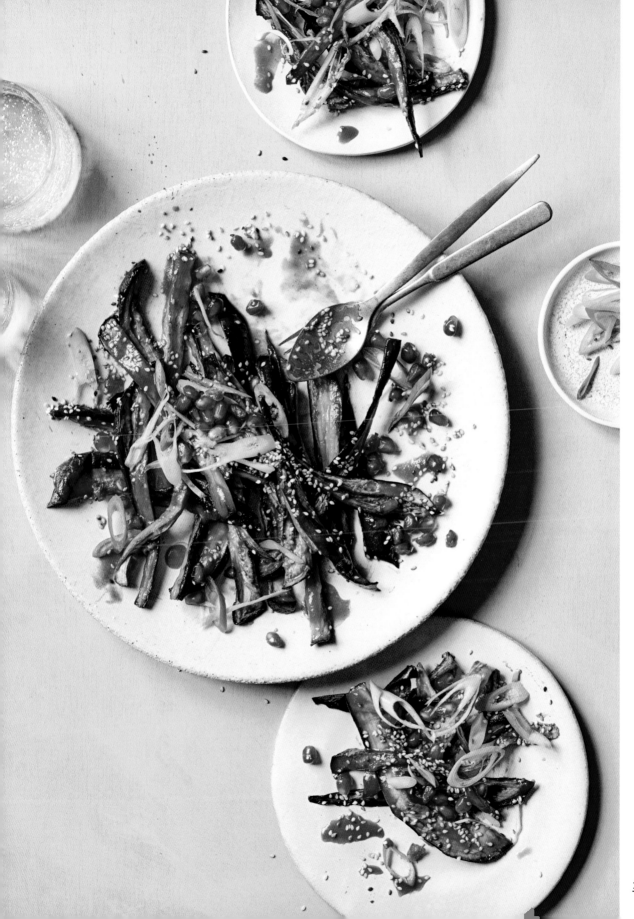

Prebiotic Tabbouleh

SERVES 4

Plant Diversity
Score: 6.25
Bonus Score: 5 or more

Many of us are, for one reason or the other, not huge fans of broccoli, cauliflower and cabbage, members of the brassica family of vegetables. There may even be a genetic reason for this, according to some studies. But even though our taste buds may not take too kindly to broccoli, our gut inhabitants love these prebiotic brassicas because they act as the perfect food for the bacteria which populate our gut microbiome.

Now, before the tabbouleh police comes out in force, I realise this is not an entirely authentic recipe. This tabbouleh has been given a revitalising gut-friendly treatment and tastes brilliant, so don't knock it until you've given it a try!

—

125g (4oz) broccoli florets

125g (4oz) cauliflower florets

50g (2oz) fine bulgur wheat, soaked in boiling water for 20 minutes

75g (2¾oz) parsley, finely chopped

15g (½oz) finely chopped mint leaves

15g (½oz) finely chopped dill

½ red onion, thinly sliced

1 tomato, finely diced

½ tsp ground allspice

Juice of 1 large lemon

2 tbsp extra-virgin olive oil

1 tsp pomegranate molasses

Salt, to taste

BONUS GUT-FRIENDLY ADDITIONS

2 tbsp toasted nuts and seeds

1 Granny Smith apple, finely chopped

½ cucumber, deseeded and finely diced

Finely diced mangetout, celery, or green beans

1. Grate the broccoli and cauliflower into a large bowl. You could also pulse the florets in a food processor, although I prefer the texture of grated.

2. Drain the bulgur and place it in the same bowl as the broccoli and cauliflower. Add the parsley, mint, dill and red onion to the bowl along with the tomato, allspice, lemon juice, olive oil and pomegranate molasses.

3. Season with salt to taste and toss everything together, adding as many of the bonus gut-friendly additions as you like. If you are not planning to eat it straight away, don't add the lemon juice until you are ready to serve.

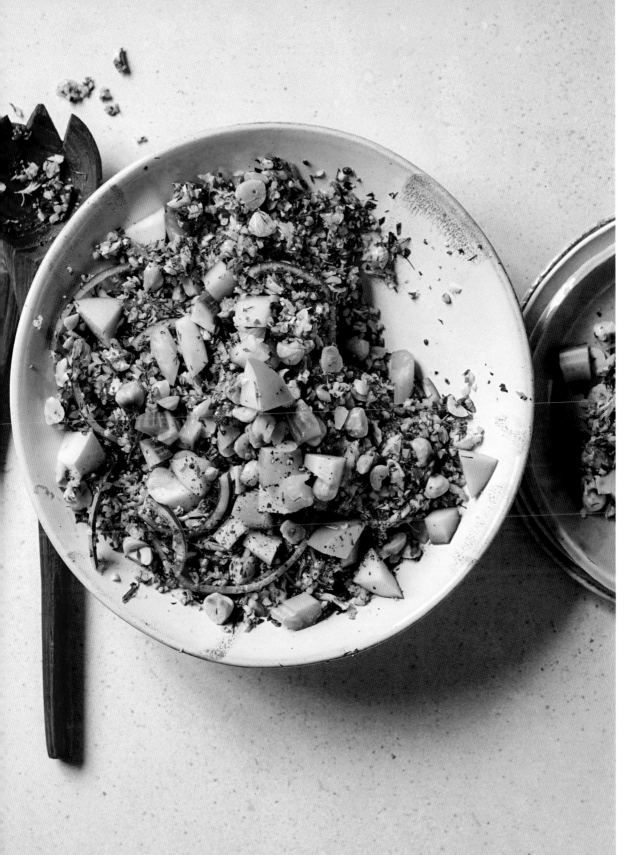

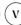 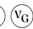

Express Hummus ①

SERVES 8

Plant Diversity
Score: 2.5
Bonus Score: 3.25 or more

If you don't have hummus on your mezze platter, then I hate to break it to you, but you don't have a mezze platter. I typically make a batch on a Monday and no matter what else I am cooking in the week, I know for a fact that this dip will be the single most popular item in our fridge. I find comfort in how easy it is to make with tinned chickpeas and how dependably it helps my gut stay healthy.

Hummus may be considered one of the most gut-healthy dips around on three accounts. Firstly, people who eat chickpeas regularly have been found more likely to have a lower weight and waist circumference, according to some large-scale population studies. Secondly, studies have shown that the fibre in chickpeas is a prebiotic which helps the beneficial bacteria in the gut multiply. Chickpeas are rich in protein and fibre, which means they release their energy slowly; steady blood sugar responses are observed after it is eaten. Thirdly, olive oil and tahini used to make hummus both contain monounsaturated fats, which are felt to be heart healthy and may also possess anti-inflammatory effects. For more on chickpeas, see page 124.

—

2 x 400g (14oz) tins chickpeas

3 small garlic cloves, roughly smashed

Juice of 1 lemon

4 heaped tbsp tahini

3 tbsp extra-virgin olive oil

Salt, to taste

TOPPINGS (OPTIONAL)

1–2 tbsp extra-virgin olive oil

1 tsp sumac

Handful of black olives

BONUS GUT-FRIENDLY ADDITIONS

Scatter the hummus with finely diced cucumber, red onion, parsley or tomato

Add 1 roasted beetroot or a handful of cooked spinach leaves to the blender when making the hummus.

1. Drain the chickpeas but retain all the water from the tin. Add the chickpeas, garlic, lemon juice, tahini, olive oil and a pinch of salt to a blender along with about 150ml (5fl oz/⅔ cup) of the aquafaba (chickpea water). Blend until smooth: if the texture is too thick, add a little more aquafaba and blend a little more.

2. Use a spatula to remove the hummus from the blender and spread it over your serving bowl. Drizzle over a little extra olive oil and sprinkle over the sumac and a few olives, and the bonus gut-friendly toppings if you like. Store in a Tupperware box in the fridge. It keeps well for 4–5 days.

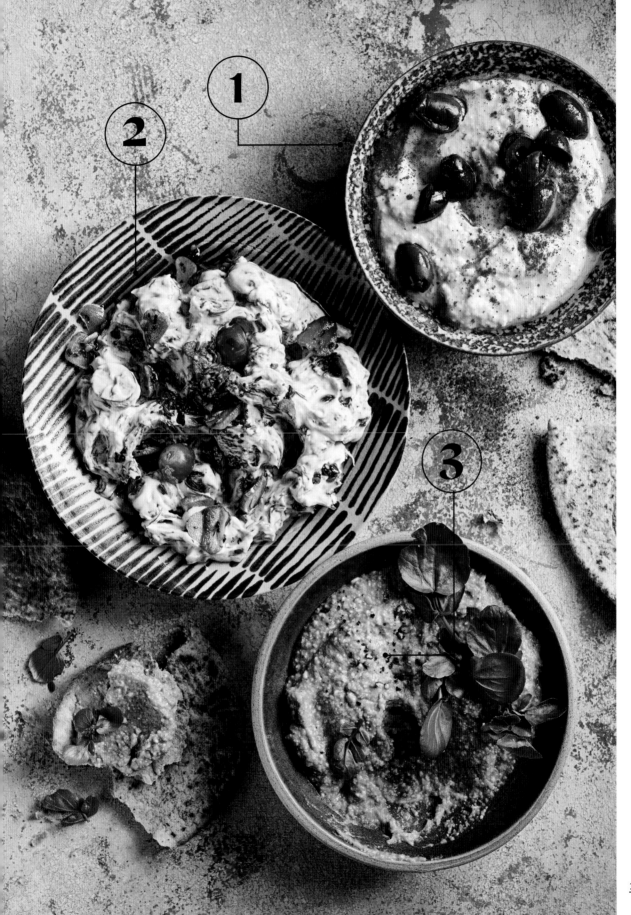

Summery Pea, Feta + Mint Dip ②

SERVES 4-6

Plant Diversity
Score: 1.75
Bonus Score: 1

325g (11oz) frozen petit pois, defrosted

200g (7oz) feta cheese

2 tbsp olive oil

1 tsp chilli flakes

Juice of 1 lime or ½ lemon

1 tsp maple syrup

Handful of mint leaves

BONUS GUT-FRIENDLY
TOPPINGS AND ADDITIONS

Handful of spinach, watercress or rocket leaves

Salty feta contrasted with sweet British peas and fresh, pungent mint is an experience you don't want to miss out on. This recipe is a great dip to serve as part of a mezze platter, or even alongside pitta crisps or tortilla chips at your next party or barbecue.

—

1. Place all the ingredients in a food processor and blitz to a smooth purée (add any gut-friendly additions here too). You can add a touch of water if necessary to help the dip come together. If the dip seems a little loose at first, don't worry – a few hours in the fridge will firm it up. Serve with a little extra crumbled feta, mint leaves, chilli and a drizzle of olive oil if you have them. It will keep in the fridge for a few days.

the kitchen prescription

Peas (Pisum sativum L.)

+ Peas are an excellent source of carbohydrates, protein and fibre. Research on the effect of peas on human heath shows that they act as prebiotics, promoting good gut health.

+ The fibre in peas helps modulate sugar responses and prevents us from becoming resistant to insulin (the hormone which controls blood

sugars and prevents diabetes).

+ Peas contain isoflavin and lectin, which help repair cells, and may have some inhibitory effects on tumour development.

+ Peas contain saponin, which is thought to reduce cholesterol through its effect on bile acids in the gut.

200

Cooling Spinach + Grape Raita

SERVES 4–6

Plant Diversity
Score: 3

I am particularly fond of this recipe, not just for its versatility but also for how inexpensive it is. With celebrity greens like kale demanding huge appearance fees and stealing the limelight, why not try some of the less glitzy greens? I use frozen spinach here; it comes compacted into little frozen spinach nuggets of goodness, which are a rather convenient addition to my freezer.

This raita is really lifted by the tadka, a technique for infusing oil with spices which adds texture and flavour to many Indian dishes.

—

300g (10oz) defrosted frozen spinach leaves

225g (8oz) natural live yoghurt or live Greek-style yoghurt (use coconut yoghurt for vegans)

Zest and juice of 1 lemon

12 purple grapes, quartered

Salt, to taste

FOR THE TADKA

2 tbsp olive oil, plus a drizzle to serve

1 tsp cumin seeds

2 garlic cloves, thinly sliced

½ tsp mustard seeds

½ tsp chilli flakes, plus a pinch to serve

1. Squeeze any extra moisture out of the spinach and place it in a bowl.

2. Heat the olive oil in a small frying pan; when hot but not quite smoking, add the cumin seeds, garlic, mustard seeds and chilli flakes. When the spices start popping vigorously and the garlic is slightly golden, pour the hot oil carefully over the spinach leaves and allow to cool.

3. Top the spinach with the yoghurt, lemon zest and juice and season with salt to taste. Stir well to combine.

4. Serve the raita in a shallow bowl topped with quartered grapes, a pinch of chilli flakes and a drizzle of olive oil. If it seems a little loose, chill in the fridge for a few hours to firm up. It keeps well in the fridge for a few days.

MEZZE

the kitchen prescription

Spinach (Spinacia oleracea L.)

+ Spinach has a diverse nutritional composition. It contains chemicals which are thought to help the body secrete hormones which both promote feelings of fullness and help control blood sugar levels.

+ Researchers have measured various heating times of spinach and their effects on the presence of the antioxidant lutein. Lutein is helpful for heart health as it dampens chronic low-grade inflammation, which can increase the risk of having heart attacks. The longer you boil spinach for, the less lutein remains and frying spinach results in all the lutein being degraded in just 2 minutes. I would suggest wilting your spinach in just a splash of water for about 1 minute in order to preserve as much lutein as possible.

Crunchy Fennel, Carrot + Halloumi Fritters with Mint Tahini Yoghurt

<u>SERVES 2</u>

Plant Diversity
Score: 4

125g (4oz) grated vegetarian halloumi

2 garlic cloves, finely crushed

75g (2¾oz) grated carrot (about 1 small carrot), moisture squeezed out

125g (4oz) finely shaved fennel

1 tsp dried mint

½–1 tsp chilli flakes

1 tsp cumin seeds

1 large egg, beaten

50g (2oz) cornflour

Salt, to taste

Vegetable oil, for frying

FOR THE MINT TAHINI YOGHURT

100g (3½oz) full-fat live Greek yoghurt

2 tbsp tahini

1 tsp dried mint

Handful of fresh mint leaves, thinly sliced (optional)

Juice of ½ lemon

There is no denying that a morsel of fried deliciousness features incredibly well on a mezze platter. While nobody here is denying the attraction of deep-fried food, there is also no escaping the fact that deep-frying as a cooking method is not the healthiest option, resulting in the absorption of significant quantities of fat. Here are my top tips to get excellent results without deep-frying:

+ Invest in an oil sprayer. This allows you to spread a thin layer of oil on to food before baking at a high temperature, therefore giving a crisp result. For optimal results you can also spray your baking paper with oil before placing the food on top of it, and then spray the food over the top.

+ Use a good-quality non-stick pan; you can then use minimal oil to still achieve a crispy golden brown result.

+ If you have space in your kitchen and can afford it, you could try an air fryer. I don't own one myself, but friends tell me it works wonders.

—

1. Combine the halloumi with the garlic, carrot, fennel, dried mint, chilli flakes, cumin seeds, egg and cornflour. Season with salt to taste and mix everything together really well. I use my hands as I think it helps break the fennel down a bit.

2. Brush just a tablespoon of vegetable oil in a medium non-stick pan and place over a medium heat. Divide the mixture into fritters – you should get about 8–10 fritters that are 5cm (2in) in diameter and 1cm (½in) thick. Fry the fritters in batches of three or four until golden; they only need 2–3 minutes on each side.

3. For the mint tahini yoghurt, mix all the ingredients together in a small bowl and serve alongside the fritters.

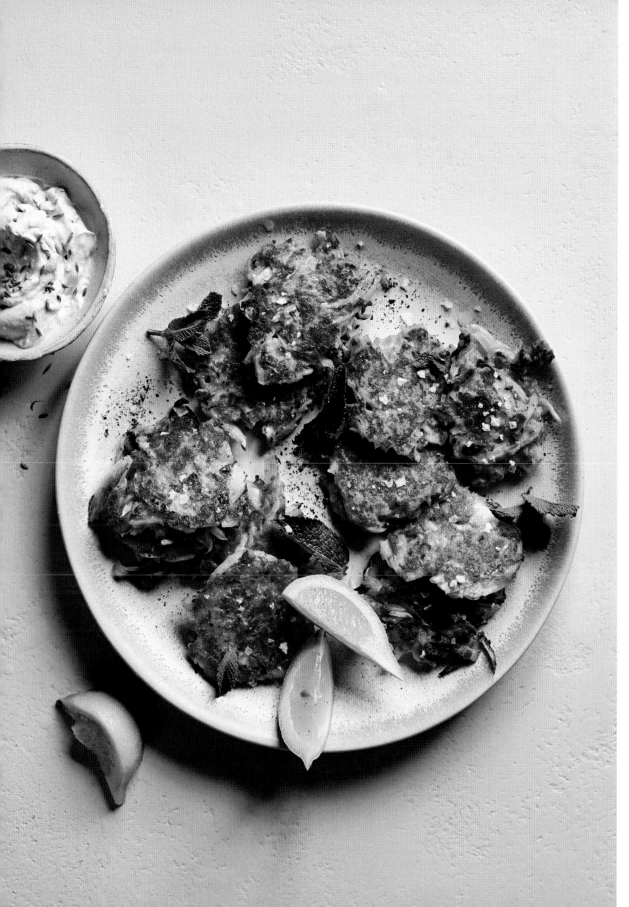

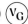

Limey Pickle Roast Cauliflower Popcorn

SERVES 4–6

Plant Diversity
Score: 2
Bonus Score: 1.25

1 tbsp lime pickle

1 tsp cumin seeds

½ tsp ground turmeric

½–1 tsp chilli flakes

2 tbsp olive oil

1 medium cauliflower (about 800g–1kg/1lb 12oz–2lb 4oz), cut into small florets

Salt, to taste

TO SERVE (OPTIONAL)

1 lime, cut into wedges

Handful of finely chopped coriander

2 tbsp live yoghurt (or plant-based yoghurt)

2 tbsp pomegranate seeds

Cauliflower is the king of cruciferous vegetables and will always hold a special place in my heart. Its status has changed of late, from the pale, sulphurous, water-logged staple of school dinners to a deeply savoury and versatile – maybe even a little trendy – brassica. These cauliflower bites are incredibly moreish, but you can use broccoli, quarters of cabbage, purple cauliflower or Brussels sprouts instead of white cauliflower if you prefer.

—

1. Preheat the oven to 220°C fan/240°C/gas mark 8 and line a large baking sheet with baking paper.

2. Mix the lime pickle with cumin seeds, turmeric, chilli flakes and olive oil to form a marinade. Pour this marinade over the cauliflower pieces and toss well to combine. Scatter the cauliflower over the lined baking sheet and season with salt to taste – you may not need much salt depending on how salty the pickle you use is. Transfer the cauliflower to the oven and bake for 20–25 minutes until the cauliflower is charred and golden.

3. Serve the cauliflower popcorn with wedges of fresh lime, coriander, yoghurt and pomegranate seeds scattered over the top if you like.

---

the kitchen prescription

Cauliflower (Brassica oleracea var. botrytis)

+ Like all cruciferous vegetables, cauliflower is a prebiotic which feeds our gut bugs, maintains the lining of the gut and improves our ability to defend against infection.

+ It contains choline, a chemical we need to make the nerve-signalling chemicals that are used in our brain.

+ Cauliflower is a source of sulforaphane, which is thought to possess some cancer-inhibiting properties.

+ Cauliflower has a plant compound called indole-3-carbinol (I3C), which acts as a plant oestrogen and may have an effect on human oestrogen regulation too.

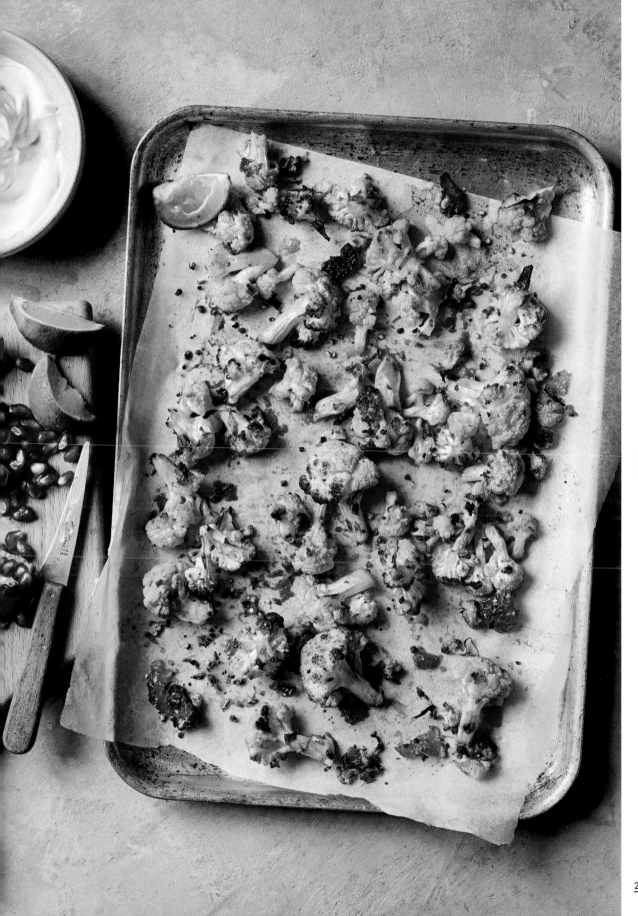

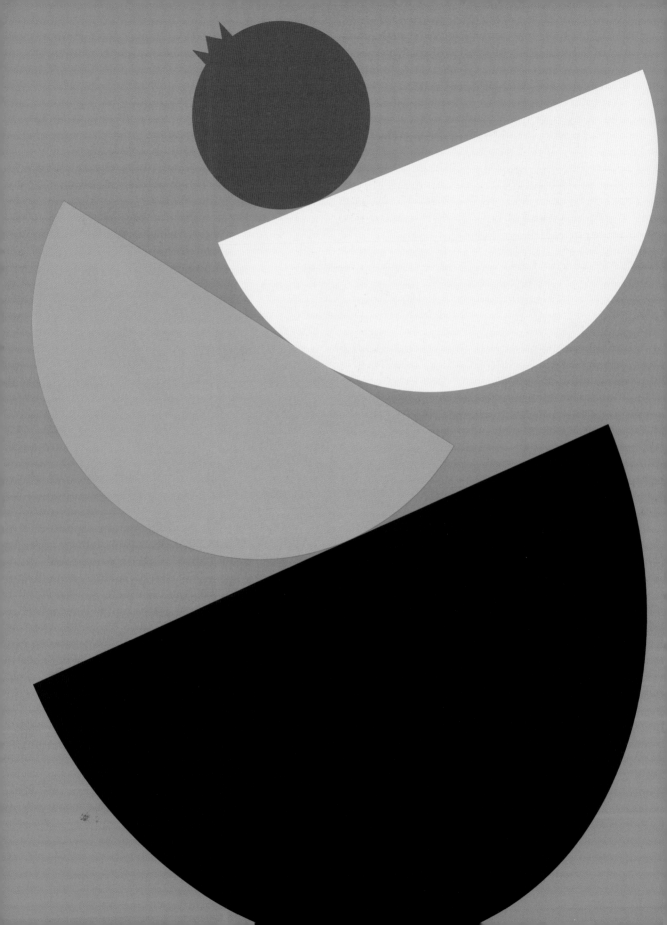

FEAST

Your gut-friendly party

Just like the act of cooking, feasting is a fundamentally human activity.

Archaeological evidence suggests that modern humans have been feasting together in many areas around the world for thousands of years. A 12,000-year-old burial cave in Galilee, for instance, has been identified as the site of the earliest feast we know about (it appears that over 70 tortoises and several butchered cattle were on the menu). Fascinatingly, these remains suggest that feasting began before the advent of agriculture; even ancient communities recognised the importance of shared eating.

Anthropologists now believe feasting to be a key characteristic of modern human society and a pivotal way to establish the cooperation necessary for humans to succeed as a species. Humans use feasts to maintain cultural systems, class systems and – in some circumstances – to compensate for the variability in availability of resources.

Fast-forward to the 21st century and transpose this innate human desire to feast against a backdrop of vast food options and excessive food availability, and it becomes clear that feasting and overindulgence have become synonymous with one another; whether in the form of sugar- and fat-laden treats, alcoholic beverages or an abundance of meat. Take it from a cookery author who is asked to write recipes for birthdays, festivals, Mother's Day, Valentine's Day and Christmas: people want extravagance on their plates more often than you would realise.

The problem this poses is that excessive feasting may affect your gut microbiome – too much of a good thing can upset the way your gut functions. Conventional indulgent party food can often lack the dietary fibre and plant-based diversity that a gut-healthy diet demands, as well as featuring an excess of saturated fats. Just think of how your belly and body feels in January after Christmas festivities: case in point.

This is where my credentials as a doctor-chef come to the fore. The recipes featured in this chapter will be the stars of your feast. They are satisfying to eat and gratifying to make, but remain totally gut-loving. In particular, in this chapter I celebrate grains, from bulgur and chickpea pilaf (page 218) to sorghum with roast radishes (page 220) and spiced roast carrots and parsnips with buckwheat (page 222).

After cooking from this chapter I want you to well and truly break away from the perception that gut-healthy foods or gut-healthy patterns of eating are just for everyday cooking, and not for special occasions. Gut-healthy foods can be indulgent, comforting, pleasuresome, satisfying, plant-centric and gut-loving all at the same time. Believe me when I say that with these feasting recipes on your table, your gut bacteria will be partying with you at Christmas, Easter, birthdays and every celebration in between.

Artichoke + Spinach Tart

Plant Diversity
Score: 3.5

When I celebrate, there is always cheese and there is always pastry. Arguably, it is hard to restore gut health with a cheese pastry, but this sophisticated pastry incorporates the goodness of nutrient-dense spinach and the prebiotic qualities of artichokes. I find jarred artichokes an essential pantry item; the marinated ones are particularly special as the flavour has seeped all the way into the flesh, but any variety will do.

—

150g (5oz) frozen spinach, defrosted

200g (7oz) ricotta cheese

1 egg, separated

1 garlic clove, grated

1 sheet of puff pastry

200g (7oz) jarred artichokes, drained from their oil

1 tbsp capers

½ tsp chilli flakes

1. Preheat the oven to 180°C fan/200°C/gas mark 6.

2. Squeeze all the moisture out of the spinach, then add to a food processor along with the ricotta, egg white and garlic. Blitz to smooth, vivid green purée. Be careful to discard the extra water that surrounds the ricotta in its packet before using it.

3. Place the sheet of puff pastry on a baking tray lined with baking paper and score the edge of the pastry all the way around to create a 2cm (¾in) border. Be careful to not score all the way through.

4. Use a spatula to spread the ricotta and spinach mixture all over the base of the tart, up to but not over the scored edges. Stud the surface of the tart with the artichokes and sprinkle over the capers and chilli flakes. Brush the edges of the pastry with the egg yolk. Transfer to the oven for 30 minutes and bake until deep golden brown. Slice into squares and serve.

the kitchen prescription

Artichoke (Cynara cardunculus var scolymus)

+ Artichokes are not actually a vegetable, but rather a type of thistle rich in fibre, folate and vitamins C and K. They are also a prebiotic.

+ Studies on artichoke extracts suggest that this thistle may lower blood cholesterol, perhaps in part because artichoke contains an antioxidant called luteolin, which evidence suggests may prevent cholesterol formation.

+ The medicinal benefits of artichoke seem to extend to the liver, particularly those with fatty livers. The antioxidants cynarine and silymarin may be partly responsible for these liver protective effects.

+ Artichokes may also help cells regenerate, although more conclusive research is needed in humans.

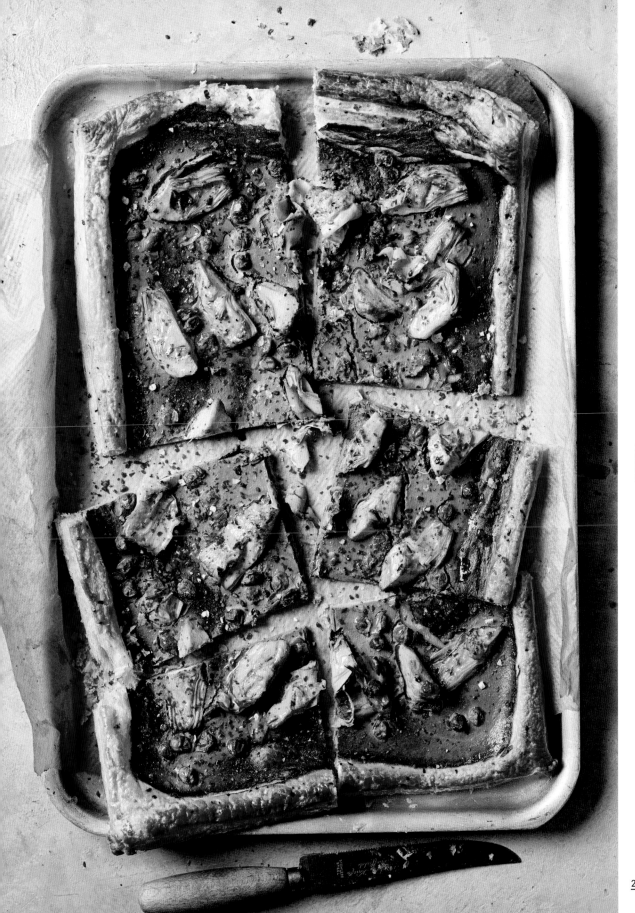

Chilli Chestnut, Sweet Apricot + Whipped Feta Toasts

MAKES 12–14

Plant Diversity
Score: 3

½ sourdough baguette

100g (3½oz) feta cheese

1 tbsp yoghurt

1 tsp olive oil

1 garlic clove, grated

180g (6oz) pre-cooked vacuum-packed chestnuts, finely chopped

1 heaped tsp harissa paste or ½ tsp red chilli paste

6 dried apricots, finely chopped

Small handful of finely chopped chives (or other herb of your choice)

Salt, to taste

Vacuum-packed, cooked and ready to eat, chestnuts have revolutionised my cooking. These fibre-dense morsels are incredibly convenient and can sit in your storecupboard for ages before you use them. I make these bite-sized toasts with this wonderful ingredient, but they can also be used for desserts at Christmas time, stuffing for roast chicken and literally hundreds of other amazing dishes.

—

1. Slice the sourdough baguette unto 1cm (½in) slices: you are looking for 12–14 slices. Place the slices of bread under a hot grill and toast for about 2 minutes on each side until the toasts are evenly golden.

2. Add the feta and yoghurt to a small food processor and blend to a smooth purée. If the mixture isn't coming together, add a tablespoon of kettle-hot water and blend again.

3. Heat the oil in a frying pan over a medium heat. Add the garlic to the oil and when it starts to turn golden, add the chestnuts and harissa and season with a touch of salt. Allow the chestnuts to heat through for a minute or two. Take the chestnuts off the heat and stir in the apricots.

4. Spread the whipped feta over the base of the toast. Sprinkle over the chestnut-apricot mixture and sprinkle over the chopped chives. Serve immediately.

the kitchen prescription

Chestnuts (nuts of the tree genus Castanea)

+ The unique soft texture of chestnuts is a result of a high water and low oil content.

+ Chestnuts are rich in fibre. This means they can act as a prebiotic, feeding our gut bacteria and in turn harbouring a healthy microbiome, as well as curbing the appetite more than other varieties of nuts.

+ They are also a rich source of polyphenols like gallic acid and ellagic acid, which may support heart health, and are thought to improve our body's response to insulin, the hormone that controls blood sugar.

+ Chestnuts are a good source of vitamin C and full of minerals like copper, potassium and manganese.

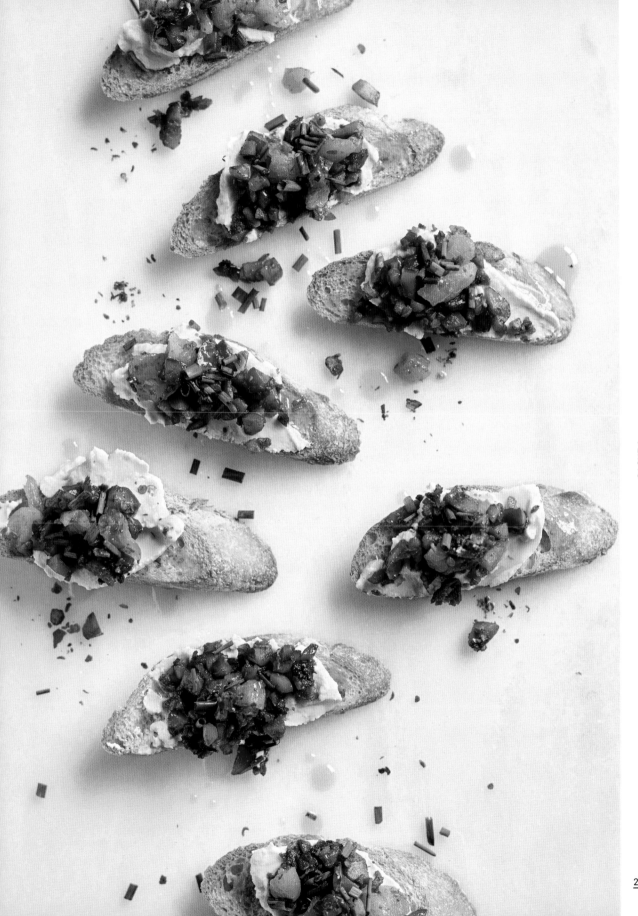

Tahini, Roast Garlic + Root Soup with Halloumi Croutons

SERVES 6

Plant Diversity
Score: 5.5
Bonus Score: 1 or more

Root vegetables are sweet, complex in their flavour profile and texture and dense with fibre – and therefore great for your gut. The addition of roast garlic and rich tahini offsets the sweetness of the root veg, creating a wonderfully complex, satisfying golden caramel-coloured soup that serves as a fantastic start to any feast.

—

2 parsnips

2 carrots

500g (1lb 2oz) swede

500g (1lb 2oz) celeriac

1 whole bulb of garlic

1 lemon, halved

2 tbsp extra-virgin olive oil

2 tbsp tahini

2 litres (3½ pints/8 cups) vegetable stock

250g (9oz) block of vegetarian halloumi cheese

1 tsp olive oil

1 tbsp toasted mixed seeds, to serve (optional)

1. Preheat the oven to 200°C fan/220°C/gas mark 7. Line a large baking tray with baking paper.

2. Roughly chop the parsnips, carrots, swede and celeriac into chunks and place on the lined baking tray. Slice off the top of the garlic bulb (horizontally) and place on the baking tray with the lemon halves and the rest of the vegetables. Drizzle the garlic bulb and vegetables with the olive oil and use your hands to rub the oil all over the vegetables. Transfer to the oven and roast for 25 minutes, or until the vegetables have started to char at the edges.

3. Place the roasted vegetables in a blender with the pulp of the roasted lemon, the garlic cloves squeezed out of their papery shells, the tahini and vegetable stock. Blitz to a smooth purée and season with salt to taste. (You may need to do this in two batches.) Transfer the soup to a saucepan, bring to the boil and then simmer for a few minutes.

4. Cut the halloumi block into 3cm (1¼in) cubes. Place a non-stick pan over a medium heat and drizzle with the olive oil. Fry the halloumi cubes for a few minutes until they are a deep golden brown colour.

5. Serve the soup with the halloumi croutons and a handful of toasted seeds, if you like.

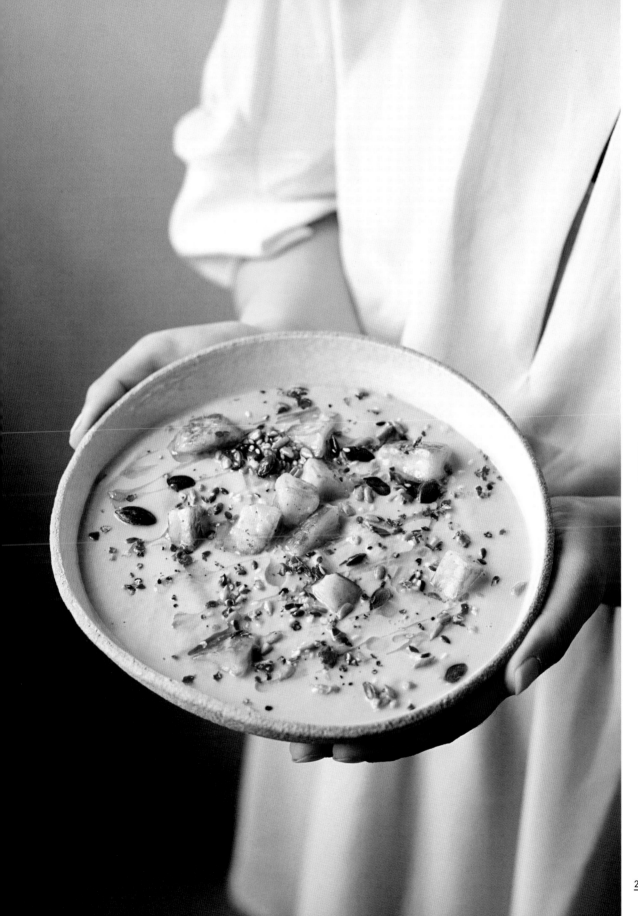

Radicchio, Plum + Seared Steak Salad

SERVES 2

Plant Diversity
Score: 2.25
Bonus Score: 1.25

It is becoming more and more important to think about how much meat we are consuming, and to begin testing the possibility that a more plant-based diet is what we need to embrace, not just for the sake of our gut, but also for the survival of our environment. But when eaten occasionally, unprocessed red meat can be a wonderful pleasure. In this recipe I have used a single steak to serve two people, although you could easily scale up to create a starter for more people. I've centred the dish around vibrant and gut-friendly radicchio and plums but feel free to experiment with other seasonal fruits and bitter leaves.

NOTE

If in season, you can use persimmons instead of plums. Or try peach, grapefruit or pomelo segments instead of plums for a change.

—

150g (5oz) radicchio

3 firm, ripe plums

1 x 200–250g (7–9oz) sirloin steak

1 tbsp vegetable oil

Flaky sea salt (I like Maldon)

FOR THE DRESSING

½ fresh red chilli, thinly sliced

1 tbsp fish sauce

1 tbsp extra-virgin olive oil

½ tsp honey

Juice of ½ lime

TO GARNISH (OPTIONAL)

Handful of fresh mint leaves

1 tbsp toasted peanuts

1. Carefully tear the radicchio leaves and place them at the base of a large platter. Using a very sharp knife, slice the plums in half, remove the stone and cut each plum half into thin slices. Place the plums in and around the radicchio leaves.

2. Rub the steak with vegetable oil and season with salt to taste. Heat a non-stick frying pan over a high heat; when it is hot but not quite smoking, add the steak. Sear it for just under 2 minutes on each side. Remove from the pan and allow to rest for 5 minutes before slicing the steak into thin strips.

3. Place all the ingredients for the dressing in a small bowl and stir well to combine. Lay the slices of steak all over the radicchio and plums and spoon over the dressing. Serve immediately, garnished with mint leaves and peanuts if you like.

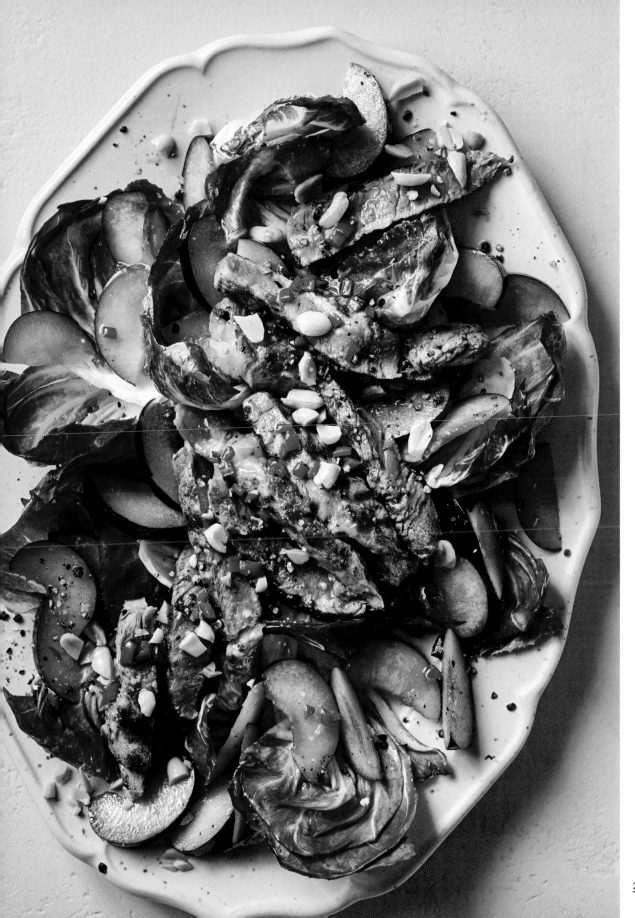

Tamarind + Ginger Charred Chicory, Bulgur Pilaf

SERVES 2–4

Plant Diversity
Score: 5.5

Chicory glazed in tart tamarind and fiery ginger is the gut-friendly star of this dish. Charring chicory on a griddle takes out the bitterness, leaving behind a warm, nutty, almost woody taste. As a side dish this recipe will pair well with a variety of indulgent mains, but it shouldn't be limited to a supporting actor role. Make more, and serve it as a showstopper in its own right.

—

2 tbsp olive oil

50g (2oz) butter

2 white onions, thinly sliced

1 tsp cumin seeds

200g (7oz/1 cup) coarse bulgur wheat

1 x 400g (14oz) tin chickpeas, drained

250ml (9fl oz/1 cup) vegetable stock

FOR THE CHICORY

4 heads of chicory

1 generous tbsp extra-virgin olive oil

2 tbsp tamarind chutney

1 tsp chilli flakes

Thumb-sized piece of ginger, peeled and grated

1 tsp honey

Handful of finely chopped parsley

Handful of finely chopped dill

Salt, to taste

1. Heat the olive oil and butter in a large saucepan, then add the sliced onions and fry over a medium-low heat for about 20 minutes. The idea is that they turn an even dark brown colour, caramelise and sweeten. Remove half the onions from the pan and set aside. Add the cumin seeds, bulgur wheat, chickpeas and vegetable stock to the onions in the pan. Stir well, place the lid on the pan and simmer over a low heat for 25 minutes until all the water is absorbed.

2. Meanwhile, prepare the chicory. Slice each chicory head in half lengthways, then brush with the olive oil and season with salt to taste. Mix the tamarind chutney, chilli flakes, ginger and honey in a small bowl. Heat a griddle pan until it is very hot. Place the chicory face down into the pan and griddle for about 4 minutes, or until the leaves are deeply charred. Turn the chicory face up and brush with the tamarind and ginger glaze. After about a minute remove the chicory from the griddle.

3. To serve, place the pilaf in the base of a serving dish and top with the chicory, the reserved caramelised onions and the herbs.

---

the kitchen prescription

Chicory (Cichorium intybus)

+ Chicory is a woody herbaceous plant in the dandelion family. The roots can be baked then ground, and used as a coffee substitute.

+ Chicory, particularly the root, is a fantastic source of inulin, a type of fibre which is beneficial to gut bacteria. Studies suggest that it can increase stool frequency and help with constipation.

+ Inulin is thought to have a beneficial effect on controlling blood sugar, particularly in diabetics.

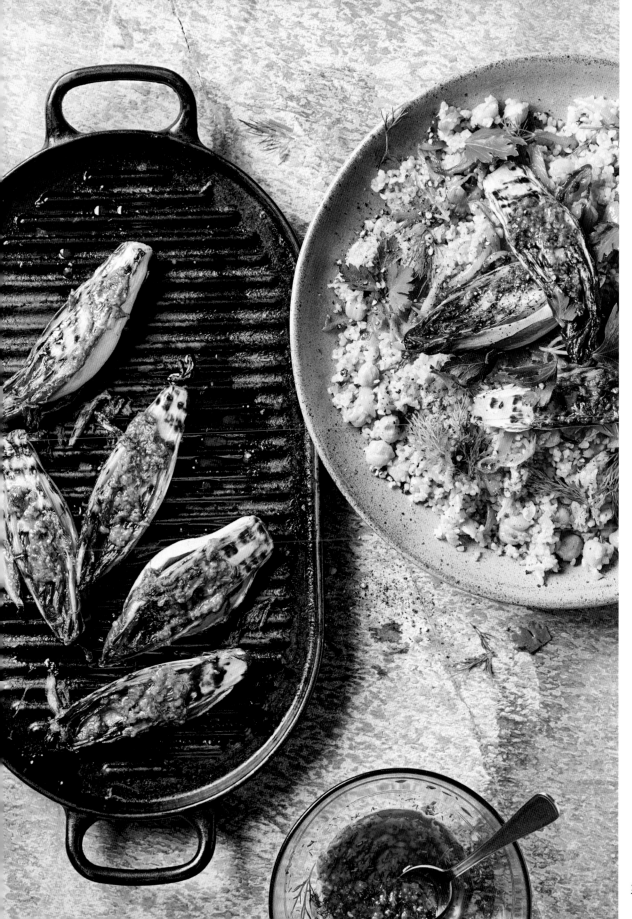

Berbere Chicken, Roast Radishes + Sorghum, Garlic Mayonnaise

SERVES 4

Plant Diversity
Score: 3.75
Bonus Score: 0.25

Berbere is a deeply evocative spice mix which forms the cornerstone of Ethiopian and Eritrean cuisine. You can make your own, but the ready-made versions are just as good. Its complex flavour profile comes from a heady mix of chilli peppers, coriander, garlic, ginger, Ethiopian holy basil seeds, korarima, rue, ajwain, nigella and fenugreek.

Sorghum, also known as juwar, is an ancient cereal grain dense in fibre and other nutrients. As it is gluten free it makes an excellent and inclusive addition to a gut-healthy feast, but if you can't get hold of sorghum, use pearl barley, bulgur wheat or freekeh instead.

—

FOR THE CHICKEN

1 medium whole chicken, skin on

6 garlic cloves

2 tbsp extra-virgin olive oil

2 heaped tsp berbere (use garam masala or ras el hanout if you can't source berbere)

1 tsp tomato purée

1 tsp honey

Juice of ½ lemon

Salt, to taste

FOR THE SORGHUM AND RADISHES

250g (9oz) dried sorghum

400g (14oz) pink radishes, halved

2 tbsp extra-virgin olive oil

1 tbsp apple cider vinegar

Few sprigs of tarragon leaves or soft herb of your choice (optional)

FOR THE MAYONNAISE

2 tbsp mayonnaise

2 tbsp full-fat live Greek yoghurt

1 garlic clove, grated

Juice of ½ lemon

1. Preheat the oven to 180°C fan/200°C/gas mark 6.

2. Start by spatchcocking the chicken: turn the chicken over so it is breast side down, then use sturdy kitchen scissors to cut down either side of the backbone. Remove the backbone, then turn the chicken over and press down firmly on the breast. You can also ask your butcher to do this for you.

3. Pound the garlic in a pestle and mortar, then mix with the olive oil, berbere, tomato purée, honey and lemon juice to form a marinade. Smother the chicken with this marinade before placing it on a baking tray and seasoning with salt to taste. Cover the chicken with foil, transfer to the oven and bake for 45 minutes, then baste with juices at the bottom of the pan and roast uncovered for another 25 minutes, or until the chicken is deep brown and the skin is crisp.

4. Meanwhile, boil the sorghum according to the packet instructions: this usually takes about 30–45 minutes. Drain, season with salt and set aside. Place the radishes on a baking tray, drizzle them with the olive oil and season with salt. Bake in the oven for 20 minutes, tossing once in between. You should be able to pierce the radishes easily with a fork and they should be golden brown. Toss the sorghum and the radishes together with the vinegar and tarragon (if using).

5. Mix the mayonnaise with the yoghurt, garlic and lemon juice. Serve alongside the chicken and sorghum radishes.

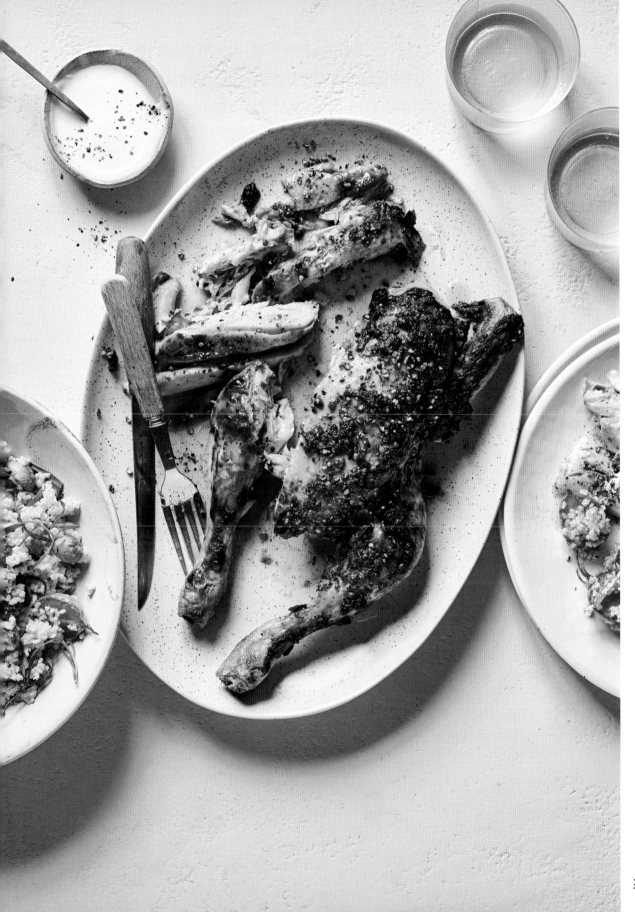

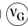

Spiced Roast Carrots + Parsnips with Buckwheat + an Olive, Pistachio + Herb Relish

SERVES 2–4

Plant Diversity
Score: 7

Roasted carrots are spiced with a fragrant spice mix from the Arabian Gulf called baharat: it includes allspice, cassia bark, cloves, cardamom and black pepper. This dish would make a fantastic accompaniment to roast turkey, turning your Christmas dinner into a gut-friendly family feast. If you can't get hold of baharat, use garam masala or ras el hanout instead. Buckwheat can also be replaced with any grain you like – try bulgur wheat, pearl barley or freekeh.

—

500g (1lb 2oz) carrots, sliced into thick batons

500g (1lb 2oz) parsnips, sliced into thick batons

1 tsp baharat

2 tbsp extra-virgin olive oil

½–1 tsp chilli flakes

½ tsp nigella seeds

175g (6oz) buckwheat

Salt, to taste

FOR THE RELISH
Handful of pitted black olives

50g (2oz) shelled pistachios

25g (1oz) parsley

1 tbsp olive oil

Zest and juice of ½ lemon

1. Preheat the oven to 180°C fan/200°C/gas mark 6 and line a large baking tray with baking paper or foil.

2. Toss the carrots and parsnips in the baharat, olive oil, chilli flakes and nigella seeds, then tip on to the lined baking tray, season with salt and transfer to the oven for 35–45 minutes, or until the vegetables are pleasantly charred at the edges. Remove from the oven and allow to cool.

3. Meanwhile, boil the buckwheat in plenty of water according to the packet instructions: this usually takes about 30 minutes. Drain, season with salt and toss the buckwheat with the roasted vegetables. Spoon on to a large serving platter.

4. Finely chop the olives, pistachios and parsley together on a wooden board. Combine with the olive oil and lemon zest and juice, then spoon this mixture over the roast vegetables and buckwheat.

the kitchen prescription

Buckwheat (Fagopyrum esculentum)

+ Buckwheat is a 'pseudocereal'; despite having 'wheat' in its name, it is actually a seed and is gluten free.

+ Buckwheat is mainly composed of carbohydrates. Evidence from animal studies suggests that the carbohydrates present in buckwheat, like fagopyritol and D-chiro-inositol, may help level out the rise in blood sugar after meals.

+ It also contains many antioxidant molecules and plant flavonoid compounds like rutin, which is thought to have beneficial effects on our health.

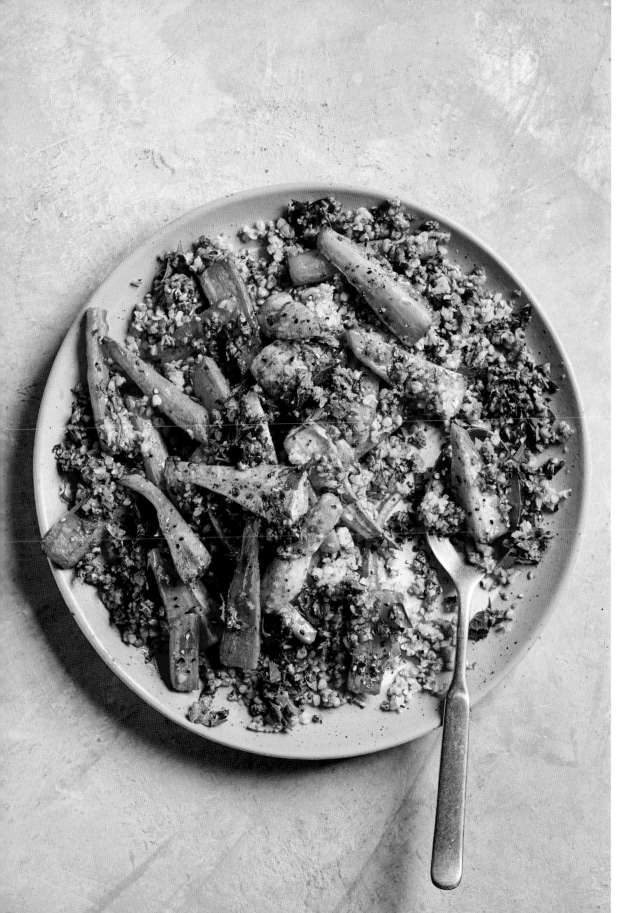

Jewelled Fennel Couscous, Slow Roast Lamb Shoulder

SERVES 6

Plant Diversity
Score: 6.5

While tender, fall-off-the-bone lamb is considered the showstopper at many a feast, this gut-friendly, fruity fennel and couscous dish easily steals the limelight from the meat. Full of herbs, nuts and dried fruit, the end result is a taste and textural joy, where the meat and the other ingredients complement each other subtly, none overpowering the dish.

—

FOR THE LAMB

1.5kg (3lb 5oz) lamb shoulder

6 garlic cloves

2 tsp red chilli paste

2 tbsp extra-virgin olive oil

1 tsp dried oregano (or a few sprigs of fresh thyme)

Generous pinch of salt

FOR THE COUSCOUS

200g (7oz/1 cup) dried giant couscous

2 fennel bulbs, sliced vertically into 1cm (½in) chunks

3 tbsp extra-virgin olive oil

50g (2oz) finely chopped dill

50g (2oz) finely chopped parsley

50g (2oz) dried sour cherries or raisins

50g (2oz) finely chopped dried apricots

50g (2oz) roughly chopped pistachios

25g (1oz) pomegranate seeds

Salt, to taste

1. Preheat the oven to 150°C fan/170°C/gas mark 3. Use a sharp knife to poke the lamb a few times to make some deep incisions which the marinade can then penetrate.

2. Bash the garlic to a paste in a pestle and mortar with a good pinch of salt. Now combine with the chilli paste, olive oil and oregano and stir well to form a marinade. Pour this marinade over the lamb and rub it all over, ensuring all of the lamb is coated. Marinate the lamb for a few hours, or ideally overnight.

3. Bring the lamb to room temperature before placing on a baking tray and covering tightly with foil. Bake in the oven for 4 hours. Remove and allow to rest for 15–20 minutes before serving.

4. Boil the couscous in salted water according to the packet instructions. Drain and set aside.

5. Place the fennel slices on a baking tray, drizzle with a generous tablespoon of olive oil and roast for 15–20 minutes until the fennel has cooked through and charred slightly at the edges. Combine the couscous with the fennel and finely chopped herbs. Gently heat the remaining 2 tablespoons of olive oil in a pan and add the sour cherries, dried apricots and pistachios to warm them through. Spoon this mixture over the couscous and scatter over the pomegranate seeds. Serve with the lamb.

Moroccan Spiced Stuffed Peppers

Plant Diversity
Score: 7

I have a bizarre obsession with stuffing vegetables, and red peppers are the most satisfying vegetable of all to stuff. The pepper's flesh scents the stuffing with the most delicious sweet juices, while simultaneously soaking up and infusing itself with the variety of flavours within the filling. It's a great way of eating more vegetables, and you can enrich the filling even further with vegetables of your choice. If you prefer, leave out the lamb and use chunks of potato or green lentils instead. I use ras el hanout here, an evocative Moroccan spice blend now readily available in most supermarkets.

—

2 tbsp olive oil

100g (3½oz) leeks, thinly sliced

1 red onion, finely diced

4 garlic cloves, finely crushed

350g (12oz) lamb mince

1 heaped tsp cumin seeds

1 heaped tsp chilli flakes

2 heaped tsp ras el hanout

1 heaped tsp smoked paprika

1 tbsp tomato purée

150g (5oz/¾ cup) medium bulgur wheat

6 large red peppers

Salt, to taste

1. Preheat the oven to 180°C fan/200°C/gas mark 6.

2. Heat the oil in a large saucepan over a medium heat. Add the leeks and onion to the oil and fry for about 7 minutes, or until the onions and leeks are softened and starting to turn golden. Add the garlic and lamb mince, turn the heat up to high and fry the lamb until the meat is a deep brown colour, this takes about 7 minutes.

3. Add the cumin seeds, chilli flakes, ras el hanout, paprika and tomato purée to the lamb and fry for a minute to release the aroma from the spices. Stir well to break down the pieces of lamb. Add the bulgur wheat to the lamb along with a cup of kettle-hot water. Bring the mixture to the boil and simmer for another 10 minutes until most of the water has evaporated. Season with salt to taste.

4. Carefully slice the top off each pepper, then stuff them with the lamb and bulgur mixture, packing it down into the peppers. Place the peppers on a deep roasting tray and pour about 100ml (3½fl oz/scant ½ cup) water into the bottom of the roasting tray. Loosely place a piece of foil over the top of the peppers and bake in the oven for 35 minutes. Remove the foil and drizzle each pepper with a little more olive oil, then return to the oven, uncovered, for a further 20 minutes until charred and jammy. Allow to cool slightly before serving.

FEASTS

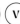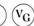

Braised Squash Masala, Herby Turnip Raita

SERVES 4–6

Plant Diversity
Score: 7.5

4 tbsp extra-virgin olive oil

2 white onions, thinly sliced

8 curry leaves (ideally fresh but can be dried)

6 garlic cloves, pound to a paste

1 tsp ground turmeric

1 tsp cumin seeds

2 tsp smoked paprika

1 tsp ground cinnamon

3–5 green chillies, finely chopped

1 x 400g (14oz) tin cherry tomatoes

3 butternut squash, peeled and cut into thick chunks (800g/1lb 12oz total weight)

Salt, to taste

FOR THE RAITA

2 turnips, peeled and chopped into large chunks

350g (12oz) natural live yoghurt or coconut yoghurt

3 tbsp finely chopped coriander

12 mint leaves, thinly sliced

1 tsp chaat masala

1 green chilli, finely chopped (optional)

Use this recipe as a template: peppers, aubergines, swede, carrots and potatoes would all work very here well instead of the butternut squash. You get a double hit of goodness here as the turnip is a brassica, making it a fantastic fibre-filled side dish when combined with herbs and yoghurt to make a raita. Use coconut yoghurt instead of live cow's milk yoghurt if you are vegan. Serve with wild rice, simple boiled grains or flatbreads of your choice.

—

1. Place a large, shallow cast-iron casserole dish over a medium heat. Add the oil and onions and sweat them for about 7–10 minutes until they are a deep golden brown, stirring frequently to ensure they colour evenly. When the onions are ready, add the curry leaves, garlic, turmeric, cumin seeds, paprika, cinnamon and green chillies. Stir well to combine, ensuring that the spices don't catch.

2. Add the tinned tomatoes to the onions and simmer for about 10 minutes, or until the mixture is well reduced and the oil starts splitting out of the sauce. Add the chunks of squash to the masala and stir well. Pour in just under a tin full of water, mix everything well and place the lid on the casserole dish. Simmer over a medium-low heat for 35–45 minutes until the extra water has evaporated away and the squash has cooked through. You may have to remove the lid for the last 5 minutes of cooking and turn up the heat to help evaporate off any extra moisture. Season to taste with salt.

3. Steam the turnips for 10 minutes, or until a knife can penetrate them easily. Allow them to cool before grating them and combining with the yoghurt, coriander, mint, chaat masala and green chilli (if using). Serve the turnip raita alongside the squash masala.

the kitchen prescription

Butternut squash (Cucurbita moschata)

+ Most people think of and cook with butternut squash as though it were a root vegetable, but technically it's a fruit that blossoms from the flower of the squash plant.

+ Butternut squash is a rich source of vitamins A and C, potassium and magnesium.

+ It contains carotenoid compounds, including beta-carotene, alpha-carotene and beta cryptoxanthin which give it a bright orange colour and are thought to be a particularly beneficial for eye health.

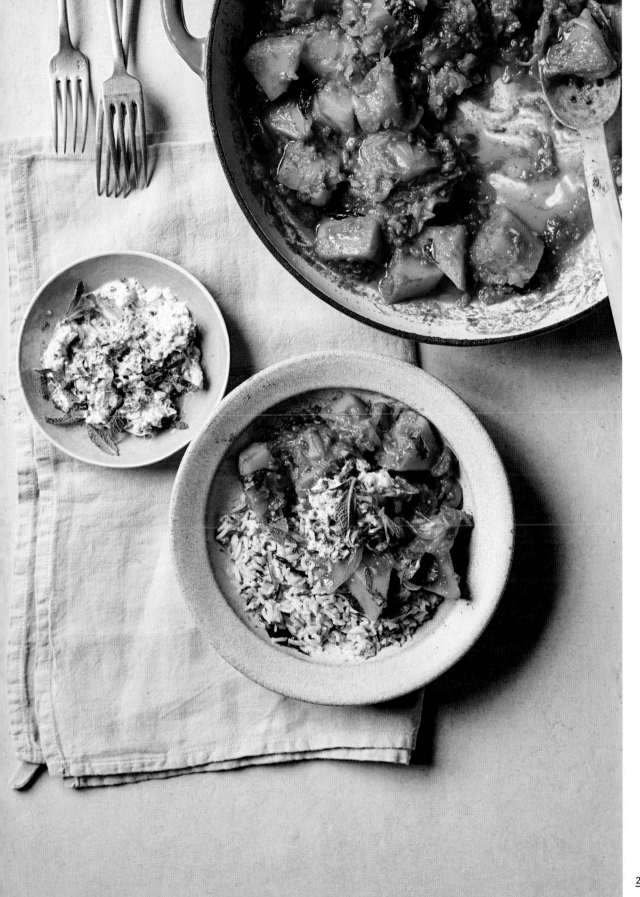

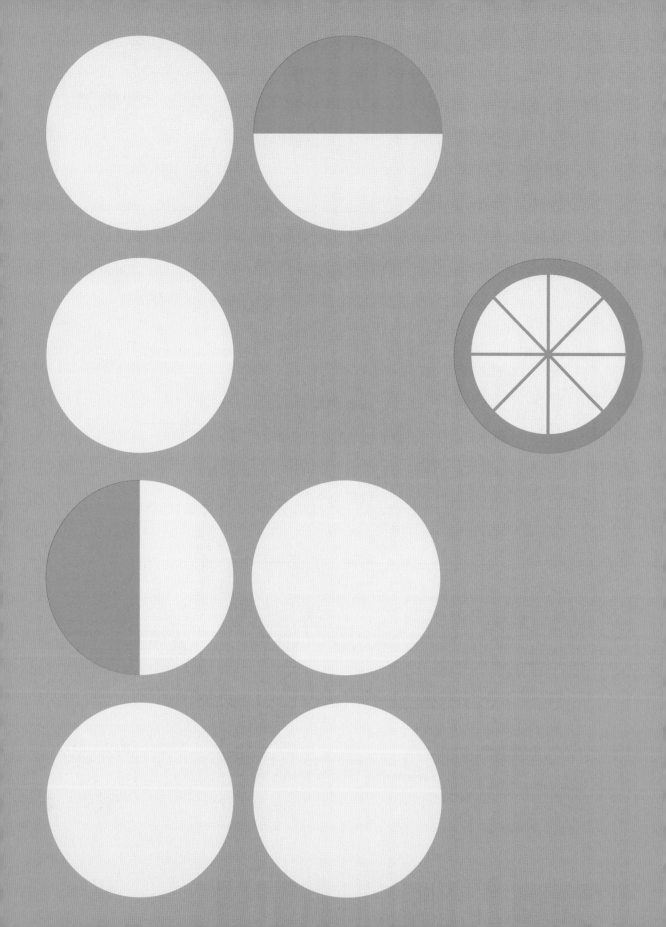

SWEET MOMENTS

Reward your taste buds AND your gut ↘

From our earliest memories, sweet is a taste we associate with happiness and celebration. There is nothing like the taste of moist chocolate cake to celebrate a special occasion, or the joy of that first lick of ice cream on a summer holiday as a child.

Sugar feeds directly into our brain's reward pathways. Different networks in the brain make up the reward system, but the key part of the brain related to craving and appetite is called the hypothalamus, a pea-sized little alcove deep in the centre of the brain. When you bite down into a jam doughnut, a chemical called dopamine is released in the hypothalamus. It sends messages to other nerves in the brain, triggering the positive emotions that we associate with chomping into that jammy delight.

From an evolutionary standpoint, we are designed to enjoy sugary foods. Our love for sweet food is so hardwired into our bodies that at around 15 weeks after conception, a foetus in the womb will swallow more sweet amniotic fluid than fluid infused with a bitter taste. Our evolutionary weakness for consuming sugar evolved in a specific set of conditions where we had to hunt to prevent starvation, and where food supplies were not always constant. Fast-forward to today and we see that there has been an exponential rise in the availability of cheap, accessible, highly processed food abundant in sugar, particularly in the last five decades.

Some scientists believe that eating certain sugary foods can be addictive. If, by eating refined sugar, we repeatedly stimulate the reward regions of the brain, this may lead to 'addictive food behaviours' or 'emotional overeating'. Studies suggest that eating sugary treats too often might interfere with how the brain processes various hormonal signals, making us feel continued cravings for the food despite having eaten enough.

Clearly, sweets are not substances of abuse like opioids, but there is some evidence of overlap in the brain circuits and molecular signalling pathways involved in sugar consumption and drug abuse. In humans, sugar can induce a release of dopamine comparable in intensity to the releases observed in the brains of people taking addictive drugs, which suggests that sugar may change the brain's reward signalling pathways in a similar way to other addictive drugs.

Given what the science is telling us about how sugar affects the brain, I feel it is important for each and every one of us to evaluate our own personal relationship with sugar. Do you turn to sugar in times of sadness, frustration, or any other heightened negative states? Are you struggling with a habitual desire to seek sweet foods for comfort?

As far as the relationship between sugar and the microbiome goes, the jury is still out on how refined sugars impact our gut bugs, although current research has shown that consuming large amounts may be harmful for the diversity of the gut microbiome. According to animal studies, high-intensity sweeteners may have negative effects on gut bugs too, but more evidence is needed to understand exactly how.

So, where does all this knowledge about the evolutionary desire and addictive nature of sugar leave us, given we are about to begin a chapter on desserts? The message from most experts is to by all means enjoy sweet foods, but in moderation. Desserts are delicious, and bring so much richness and colour to our lives and no amount of science can detract from this fact or fight our evolutionary urge to order the occasional sweet treat after dinner.

However, this chapter is called Sweet Moments for a reason. Eating desserts should be a special event, a moment of joy, a celebration, associated with feasting, family, friends and festivity, not an everyday occurrence. I have designed recipes with gut health in mind, full of probiotics like kefir, kombucha, labneh and plenty of fruits, nuts and seeds. Dark chocolate makes an appearance, as does nature's favourite dessert item, dates. I hope that through these dessert recipes you can satisfy your craving for something sweet but also come closer to achieving a sense of digestive health and happiness.

Nutty Coffee Mascarpone Stuffed Dates

SERVES 4

Plant Diversity
Score: 3

1 tsp good-quality instant coffee powder

140g (4½oz) mascarpone, chilled

500g (1lb 2oz) Medjool dates

Generous handful of roasted whole almonds

50g (2oz) melted dark chocolate

2 tsp edible dried rose petals (optional)

Here creamy, coffee-spiked mascarpone pairs perfectly with crunchy roast almonds and sweet, nutrient-dense dates. You can use any nuts, such as pistachios or pecans, and feel free to substitute the coffee for any other flavourings of your choice, for example vanilla extract, orange blossom water or rosewater.

—

1. Dissolve the coffee in a few teaspoons of boiling water and pour this concentrated coffee paste on to the mascarpone cheese. Mix the coffee into the mascarpone using a small whisk.

2. Carefully make a lengthways incision in each date and pop out the stone. Use a teaspoon to stuff the dates with the coffee flavoured mascarpone. Then stud an almond or two into the mascarpone filling. Arrange the dates on a serving platter, then drizzle with the dark chocolate and decorate with a few dried rose petals (if using). Chill in the fridge for 30 minutes or so before serving. They will keep in the fridge for a few days.

Coffee

+ Many of us rely on a strong cup of coffee to get us going in the morning (in more ways than one, if you catch my drift). The good news is that there is now evidence that coffee might be good for our gut health.

+ A diverse microbiome is considered a healthy microbiome, and coffee drinkers seem to have higher microbiome diversities. This might be because coffee is full of polyphenols and soluble fibre compounds that feed our beneficial gut microbes and increase their diversity and activity.

+ There are more than a thousand different bioactive molecules in coffee, so it is no surprise that coffee has been linked to a reduced risk of diabetes, heart disease, Parkinson's disease. Alzheimer's disease and various types of cancer.

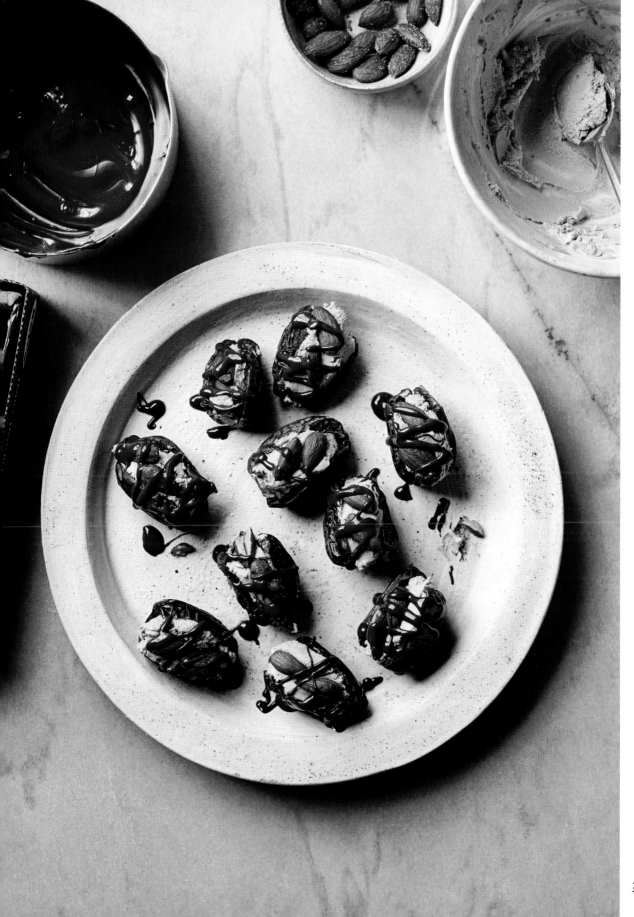

Labneh, Passion Fruit + Ginger Cheesecake

Plant Diversity
Score: 2

The classic cheesecake has been given a gut-healthy makeover: the ginger base contains toasted gut-friendly seeds, the filling is made with labneh, and it's adorned with seedy, fibrous jewels of tart passion fruit. A showstopper if there ever was one, and the bonus is there's no baking required.

—

FOR THE BASE

250g (9oz) ginger nuts

100g (3½oz) mixed seeds, toasted

125g (4oz) melted butter

FOR THE FILLING

200g (7oz) white chocolate

200ml (7fl oz/generous ¾ cup) double cream

600g (1lb 5oz) labneh (or full-fat cream cheese)

1 tbsp honey

Seeds and juice of 8 passion fruit

1. Start by lining the base of a 23cm (9in) springform cake tin with baking paper.

2. Blitz the ginger nuts and half the mixed seeds in the blender to form fine crumbs. Add the rest of the toasted seeds to the blitzed biscuits, along with the melted butter, and stir well. Press the mixture into the bottom of the lined tin, ensuring that you work the crumb evenly all the way to the edges. Chill the base in the fridge while you make the filling.

3. Melt the white chocolate in the microwave in 30-second bursts and allow to cool slightly. (Alternatively, break the chocolate into a heatproof bowl and set over a pan of simmering water until melted.) Whip the cream in a bowl using an electric whisk until it has firm peaks.

4. In a separate bowl, whisk the labneh and honey together for just a minute until smooth. Now fold the double cream and labneh together, ensuring they are well combined. Add the cooled melted white chocolate and whisk for just a minute to mix everything together evenly.

5. Spread this cheesecake mixture on to the prepared biscuit base, making sure you work your way to the edges and that there are no gaps. Smooth the surface as best you can with a palette knife and transfer the cheesecake to the fridge for 8–10 hours, or ideally overnight.

6. To serve, remove the cheesecake from the springform tin and slide it carefully off the paper on to a serving dish. Top with the passion fruit seeds and juice, or any other fruit you like. Any leftovers will keep in the fridge for a couple of days.

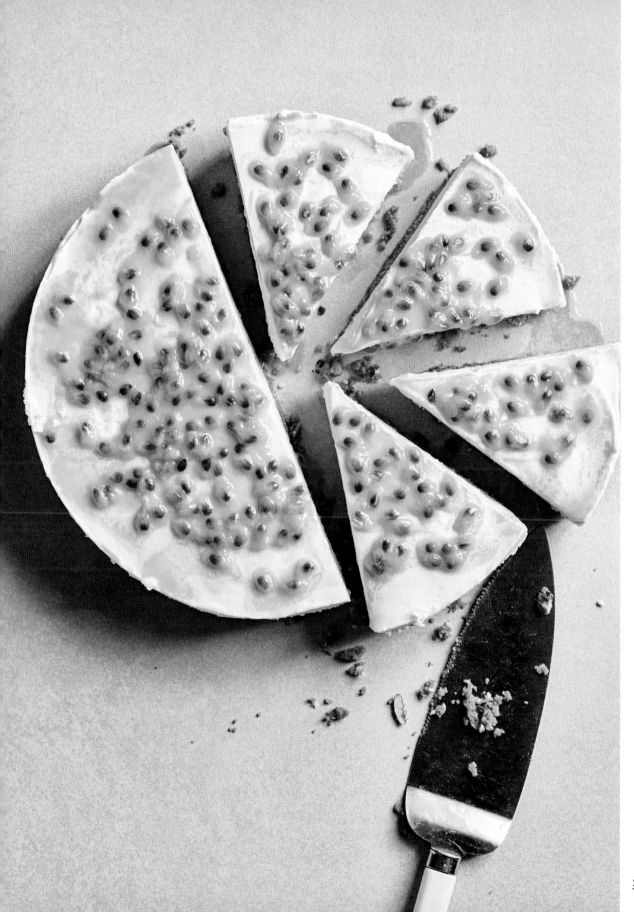

Strawberry, Sumac + Turkish Delight Ice Cream

SERVES 2 GENEROUSLY

Plant Diversity
Score: 1.25

I am a huge fan of this recipe on many accounts. Firstly, it takes less than five minutes to prepare and does not need to be churned. Secondly, it is cost-effective given that it uses frozen berries (which are both fibre-dense and nutrient-rich) and live probiotic Greek yoghurt. Thirdly, it taste utterly fantastic: sherbet-y, intensely fruity, sorbet-like, tart with chewy bits of rosy Turkish delight to finish. I could go on and on rambling about its merits, but perhaps it's best I just let you try it for yourself.

—

500g (18oz) frozen strawberries

350g (12oz) full-fat live Greek yoghurt

2 tbsp pomegranate molasses

2 tbsp sumac

4 tbsp honey or maple syrup

12 squares of Turkish delight, roughly chopped

1. Place all the ingredients, except for the Turkish delight, in a high-speed blender or good-quality food processor. Start the blender on the lowest speed, then quickly increase to the highest speed, stopping to push the ingredients down and then blending again. If the mixture is just too firm, add a tablespoon more yoghurt, or a splash of milk.

2. In about 30–60 seconds, the sound of the motor will change, and 4 mounds should form. Stop the machine. Do not overmix or the mixture will start to melt. Remove the ice cream from the blender and scoop it into bowls. Scatter over the Turkish delight and serve immediately. If the mixture appears too loose, transfer to a freezer and allow it to firm up a little before serving.

the kitchen prescription

Sumac (Rhus coriaria)

+ Sumac is a variety of flowering shrub related to the mango and cashew family of trees. There are over 200 different species of sumac, but the one used in our kitchens is called Syrian sumac.

+ The nutrient profile of sumac is not completely understood, but some early research shows that a fifth of it is made of fat, particularly oleic

and linoleic acid, which are associated with good heart health.

+ There is speculation that sumac may have sugar-lowering, antimicrobial and antifungal properties.

+ Sumac works incredibly well in desserts as well as on salads or as a hummus topper. Malic acid gives it its classic tart flavour.

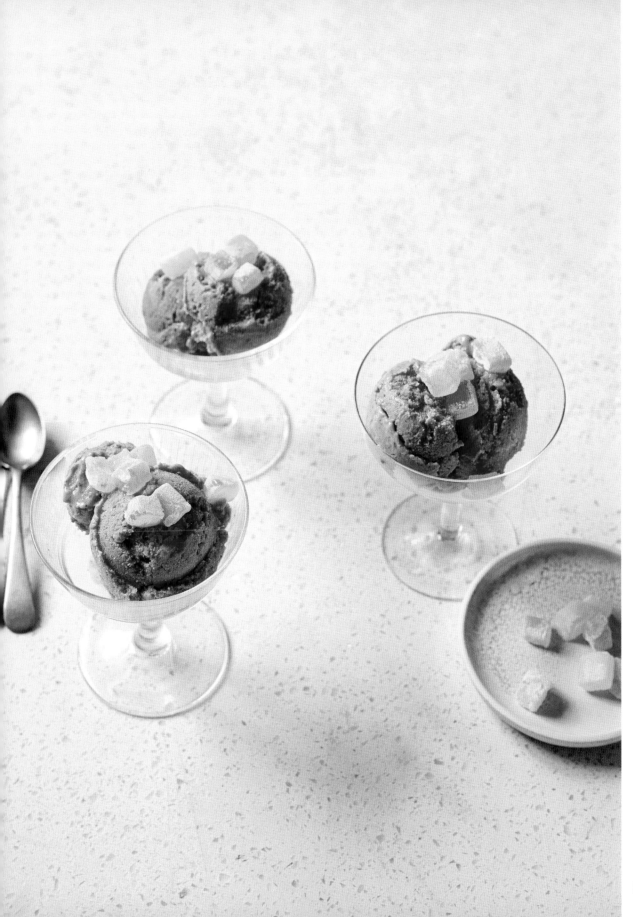

Refreshing Citrus Platter with Star Anise Syrup

SERVES 4

Plant Diversity
Score: 2.75

This is one of the easiest and most refreshing desserts around. Sliced rounds of oranges and grapefruit are drizzled with sweet spiced fennel and star anise syrup. The recipe does make more syrup than you need, so you can keep the extra syrup in your fridge to top Greek yoghurt and fruit for breakfast the next day.

—

200g (7oz) powdered jaggery (or soft light brown sugar)

2 star anise

1 tbsp fennel seeds

4 cardamom pods, bashed

4–6 large oranges (or use blood oranges or grapefruit)

1. Put the jaggery, star anise, fennel seeds and cardamom pods into a saucepan with 500ml (17fl oz/2 cups) water and bring to the boil. Simmer for about 20 minutes until the mixture starts looking a little thicker. Strain through a sieve and allow the syrup to cool. It will thicken as it cools – you are aiming for a sticky, maple syrup-like consistency.

2. Using a sharp knife, carefully slice off the top and bottom of each orange. Using even downward strokes, slice the skin away from the flesh and discard, including any remaining white pith. Turn the orange on its side and slice it into 1.5cm (⅝in) thick slices. Arrange these slices on a platter, drizzle over a few tablespoons of the syrup and serve.

the kitchen prescription

Oranges (Citrus sinensis)

+ Most of us already know that oranges are an excellent source of vitamin C, which helps support the immune system.

+ The vitamin C and citric acid present in oranges actually helps the absorption of iron in the gut. So, if you are anaemic, it is well worth taking your iron tablets with an orange.

+ Oranges contain hesperidin and naringenin, two flavonoid compounds that act as antioxidants in the body, preventing cells from damage. They may exert a beneficial effect on blood lipids and blood glucose too.

+ To get the maximum beneficial fibre from oranges, eat the whole orange rather than just drinking the juice.

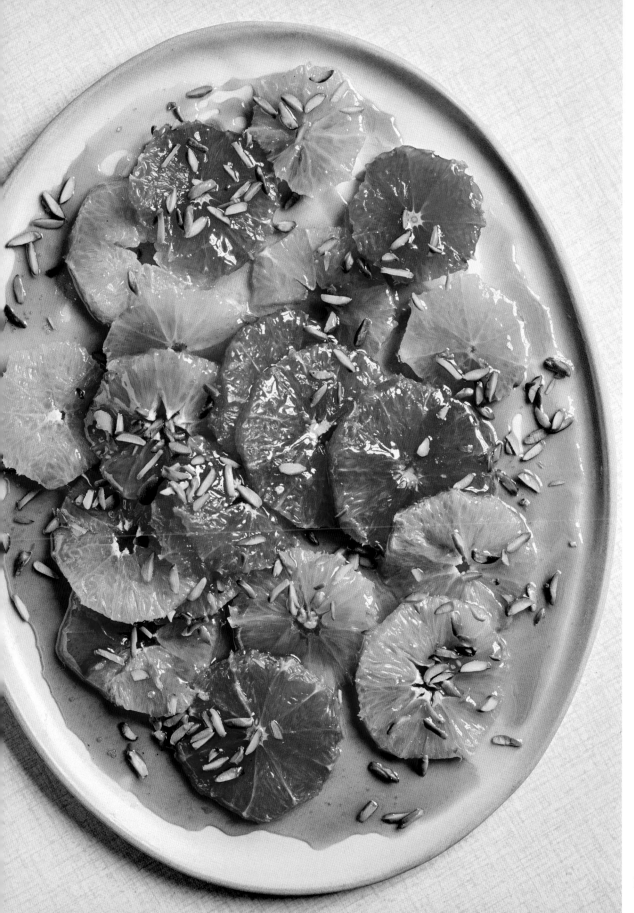

Blackberry Kefir Panna Cotta with Toasted Almonds

SERVES 4

Plant Diversity
Score: 2

Wibbly wobbly panna cotta. So often people are scared to make panna cotta until they realise just how easy it is. I use kefir here; it has a tart, lactic tang like buttermilk and a slight fizz due to the presence of carbon dioxide, an end product of the fermentation process.

Kefir pairs beautifully with sweet, tart British blackberries, though you can use any summer fruit of your choice. In this recipe, the gelatine is dissolved in hot double cream, which is then cooled slightly before the kefir is added; this stops the kefir from reaching a high enough temperature for all the good bugs proliferating within it to denature (fingers crossed).

—

350g (12oz) blackberries, plus extra to serve

250ml (8fl oz/1 cup) kefir

150ml (5fl oz/⅔ cup) double cream

100g (3½oz) powdered jaggery (or soft light brown sugar)

3½ sheets of platinum-strength gelatine

50g (2oz) toasted flaked almonds

1. Place the blackberries in a saucepan with 100ml (3½fl oz/scant ½ cup) water and simmer over a medium heat for 5–7 minutes to soften the berries and break them down to a pulp. Pass this pulp through a sieve to extract the sweet blackberry juice (discard the seeds). Allow the blackberry juice to cool before stirring through the kefir: this is a most satisfying thing to do and results in the most gorgeous mauve colour.

2. Heat the double cream and jaggery in a clean saucepan over a low heat until just at boiling point. Remove from the heat and allow to cool slightly.

3. Soften the gelatine by soaking it in some warm water. When it is very soft, squeeze out the moisture and drop it into the warm cream mixture. The gelatine should dissolve immediately; if it doesn't, place over a very low heat until it does.

4. Once the gelatine has dissolved in the double cream, allow it to cool for a minute before stirring through the blackberry kefir mixture. Pour the panna cotta mixture carefully into 4 individual ramekins or dariole moulds. Transfer to the fridge to set for at least 6 hours, ideally overnight.

5. If you have used dariole moulds, dipping each one in boiling water for 10 seconds before turning out the panna cotta will help to detach it easily. (If you've made these in ramekins, just serve them in the ramekins.) Serve topped with toasted flaked almonds and a few extra blackberries.

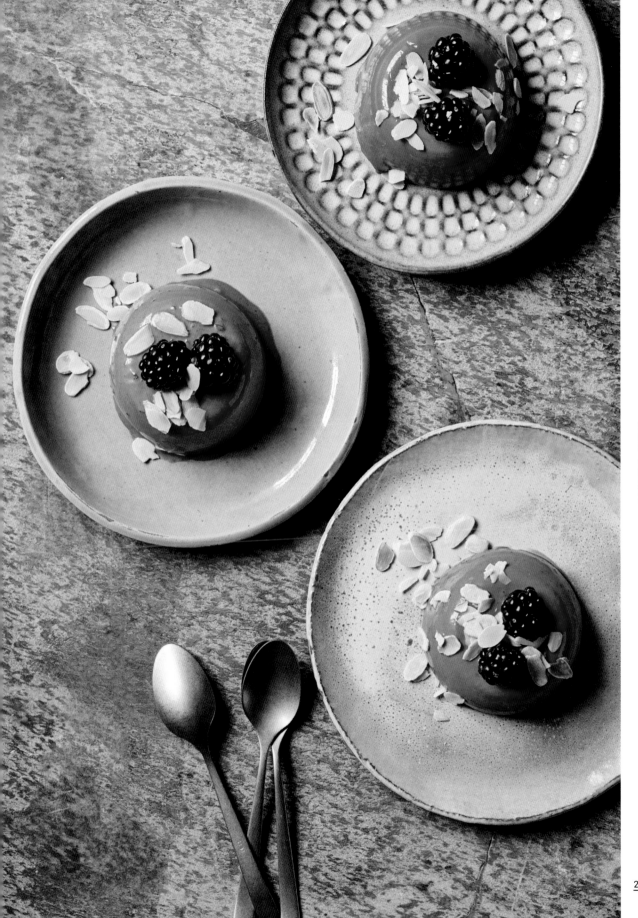

Gutlicious Rocky Road

Plant Diversity
Score: 4.25

A bite of chocolate is possibly the most cheerful, reassuring, soothing and uplifting thing in the whole world. Thankfully dark chocolate is also very good for your gut, so (dark) chocolate escapism is allowed once in a while. It's especially good when combined with fibre-dense dried fruit and nuts, as in this recipe for rocky road. It's a real treat at the end of a meal, served with a strong cup of coffee.

—

175g (6oz) dark chocolate

125g (4oz) date molasses

5 digestive biscuits

5 dried figs, roughly chopped

50g (2oz) dried apricots, roughly chopped or jumbo green raisins

50g (2oz) sour cherries

75g (2¾oz) shelled pistachios, toasted

1 tbsp cocoa powder

1. Start by lining an 18cm (7in) square tin with baking paper. Break the dark chocolate into pieces and put into a heatproof bowl set over a saucepan of simmering water (make sure the base of the bowl doesn't touch the water). Melt the chocolate, stirring occasionally, then remove it from the heat and stir in the date molasses.

2. Crush the biscuits so they are a mixture of rubble and larger pieces. Add the crushed biscuits to the melted chocolate along with the figs, apricots, sour cherries and pistachios. Stir everything well with a wooden spoon to combine and tip into the lined tin. Spread and press the mixture into the corners, then transfer to the fridge and chill for a few hours.

3. To serve, dust the surface with cocoa power and then cut into about 8–12 pieces. Store in an airtight container for a couple of days.

the kitchen prescription

Chocolate (Theobroma cacao)

+ Cocoa comes from the roasted and ground pods of the cacao tree, otherwise known as Theobroma cacao, which translates as 'food for the Gods' in Greek.

+ The percentage of cocoa in dark chocolate is important – choose an organic brand that is at least 70 per cent cocoa solids to get maximum natural fibre, minerals, vitamins and antioxidants and minimum refined sugar and additives. Fun fact: chocolate

has several times more antioxidants than green tea or red wine.

+ There is evidence that the polyphenols and flavonoids in dark chocolate boost beneficial gut bacteria (prebiotics), improve heart health, decrease cholesterol levels, positively impact mood and brain function, moderate insulin production and sensitivity and even promote healthier skin.

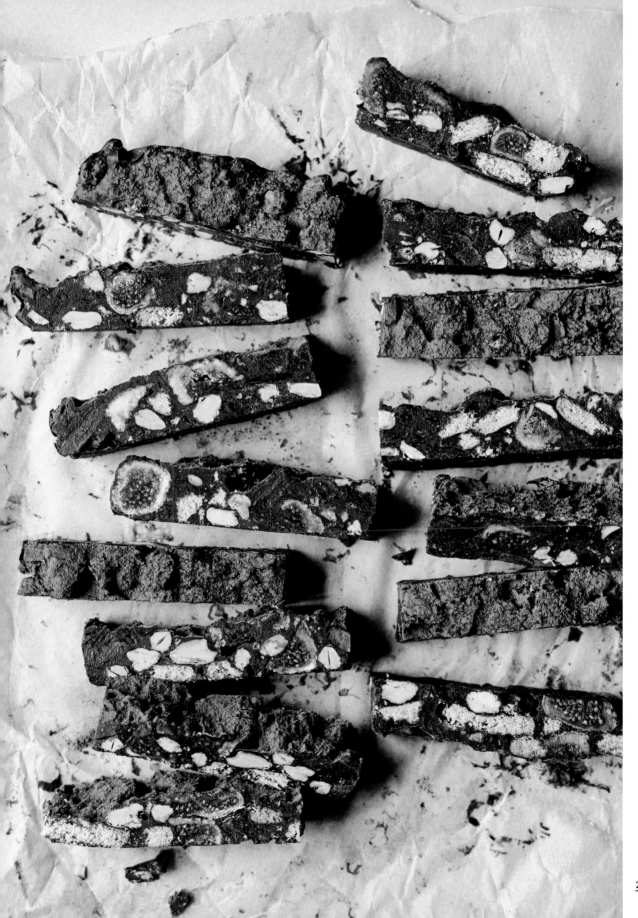

Kombucha, Raspberry + Elderflower Jelly

Plant Diversity
Score: 1

2 x 275ml (9fl oz) bottles of raspberry and elderflower kombucha (or plain kombucha with 2 tbsp elderflower cordial)

1–2 tbsp honey

5 leaves of platinum-strength gelatine

175g (6oz) fresh raspberries

An elegant, wobbly, slightly fizzy raspberry-studded masterpiece: more packed with berries than your usual jelly, but this is deliberate, given the fact that raspberries are one of the most fibre-dense fruits around.

—

1. Pour one bottle of the kombucha into a saucepan and add the honey. Bring this to the boil and then remove from the heat. Allow the kombucha to cool slightly before adding the gelatine leaves; leave them to dissolve into the hot kombucha, stirring well to ensure everything is well combined.

2. Add the second bottle of kombucha and the raspberries to the dissolved gelatine mixture and stir well. Pour the mixture into a medium jelly mould and chill in the fridge for 12 hours, or ideally overnight. It does take quite some time to set this particular jelly.

3. To remove the jelly from the mould, dip it for a few seconds in boiling water before turning out on to a serving plate.

---

the kitchen prescription

Kombucha

+ Kombucha is a slightly effervescent, sweetened black or green tea drink that has been around for thousands of years and is considered a probiotic. It often has added flavourings, for example, rose, ginger or juniper.

+ During the fermentation process bacteria and yeast form a mushroom-like film on the surface of the liquid, which is why it is sometimes called 'mushroom tea'. The fermentation process produces acetic acid, trace alcohol and gases that make the kombucha carbonated.

+ There are virtually no studies looking at its beneficial effects in humans, though animal studies indicate that it may be helpful in lowering cholesterol and protecting the liver from toxicity and improving blood sugar levels.

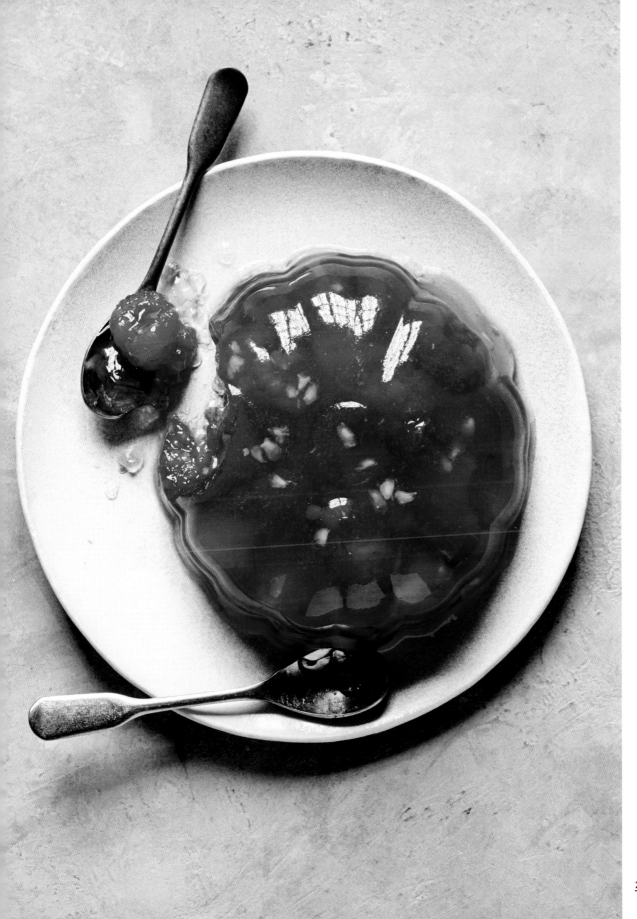

Honey-glazed Bananas with Toasted Pecans + Goats' Cheese

Plant Diversity
Score: 2.25

Bubbling hot honey-sweetened bananas with a crack of black pepper and the salty fresh tang of probiotic goats' cheese: this is a match made in culinary heaven, and is terribly easy to put together, too.

—

4 large unripe bananas

4 generous tbsp honey

½ tsp coarse black pepper

50g (2oz) toasted pecans, roughly chopped

200g (7oz) vegetarian goats' cheese

BONUS GUT-FRIENDLY ALTERNATIVES

Use hazelnuts, macadamia nuts, Brazil nuts or pistachios instead of pecans

Live yoghurt, labneh or crème fraîche would make good alternatives to goats' cheese

Switch to maple syrup and coconut yoghurt for a vegan alternative

1. Preheat the grill to a high setting. Line a baking tray with baking paper.

2. Peel the bananas and then slice them in half lengthways. Lay them on the baking tray, flat side facing upwards. Drizzle the honey over the bananas using a teaspoon and then sprinkle over the black pepper.

3. Transfer to the grill for 4–6 minutes, or until the honey is bubbling and starting to turn golden (they can burn easily, so be wary). Serve 2 slices of banana per person with the toasted pecans scattered over the top and the goats' cheese next to the warm bananas.

the kitchen prescription

Bananas (Musa sapientium)

+ A banana consists almost entirely of carbohydrates and water: it actually holds very little protein and no fat.

+ Green, unripe bananas are full of resistant starches, a type of indigestible fibre that acts as a prebiotic for gut bacteria. As the banana sits in your bowl forgotten, it ripens and becomes sweeter, and its fibre content decreases.

+ Bananas may help support our mood: they contain tryptophan, an amino acid that the body converts to the feel-good brain chemical 'serotonin'.

+ Unripe bananas may help neutralise stomach acid: a plant compound in bananas called leucocyanidin might even improve the thickness of the mucous layer in the stomach – handy if you suffer with heartburn.

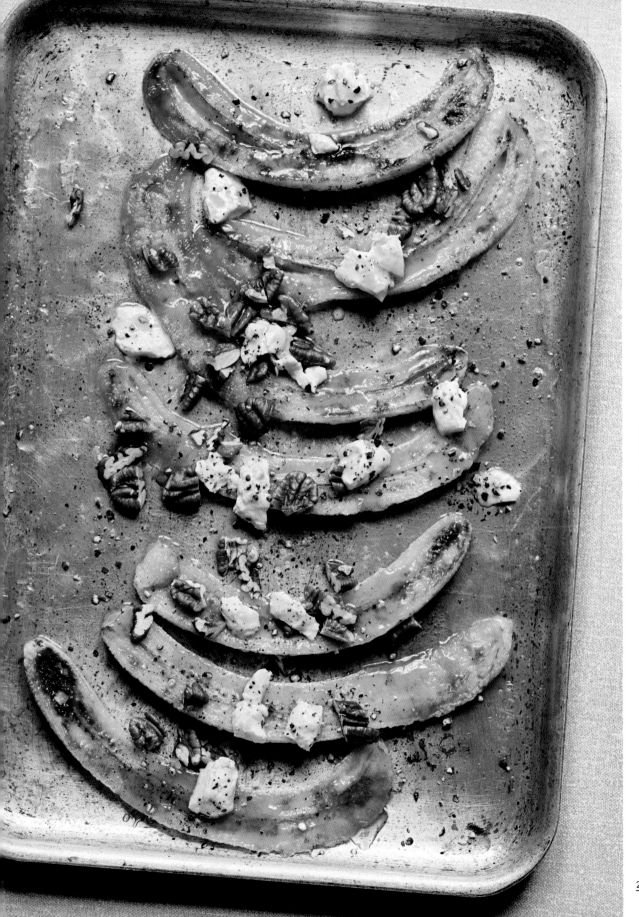

Index

Thank You

Although it is my name that finds itself on the cover of this book, there is no denying that the gruelling hard work required to make this cookbook a reality is not mine alone. I have a multitude of people to thank for their selfless contributions to *The Kitchen Prescription*.

First and foremost, my editor Nicky Ross and literary agents Heather Holden Brown and Elly James. These three ladies are my superheroines, a fantastically powerful trio. When I put pen to paper, it is their unwavering faith in my abilities as a chef and scientist that drives me to be the very best version of myself. Their complete honesty and constructive critique has shaped this text for the better in more ways than anyone can imagine.

I would also like to extend my thanks to all my close family and friends who have joined me on my 'Kitchen Prescription' journey. To my husband, whose gut is the primary subject of all my kitchen experiments, I love you! Thank you for being so open to trying the gut friendly way of life.

Thanks also to Aunty Safiya who has been my devoted kitchen assistant while recipe testing. Without your help sorting things into endless tupperware boxes, doing dishes, cleaning surfaces and sorting cupboards, I would have lost my marbles multiple times over. Sheriar Arjani my friend and writing companion, thank you for hours and hours of your precious time. It is your graft that has helped me make *The Kitchen Prescription* an accessible text, with the ability to tangibly influence people's lives.

Nikki Dupin and Emma Wells and the outstanding team at Studio Nic&Lou are the powerhouses who have designed *The Kitchen Prescription*. Words are not sufficient to explain how much love I have for these women. Thank you for understanding my vision and making it a reality so gracefully. Steve Joyce on photography: what a dream you are my friend! When I look at all the photographs in this book I am struck not just by how crisp, colourful and joyous they look, but they also take me back to those happy moments where they were captured in your studio.

Thank you to the wonderful Isabel Gonzalez-Prendergast for your exceptional organisation and positivity as Project Editor. You really are instrumental to the success of this book. My sincerest thanks to the wonderful Olivia Nightingall for all her efforts pushing this text to the finish line. Thank you dear Lizzie Harris (food styling) and Max Robinson (prop styling) for your effortless artistry and natural ability to capture beauty: I am eternally in awe. A huge thank you also to all the sales, marketing, publicity and rights teams at Hodder and Stoughton who work instrumentally behind the scenes to make this book a success.

Finally, I would like to thank all those healthcare professionals, scientists, doctors and dieticians who ask the question 'what should I eat for good gut health?' every day. Even in times of difficulty, please don't ever lose faith in your scientific endeavour. It has the power to impact individuals' lives in a way that nothing else really can.

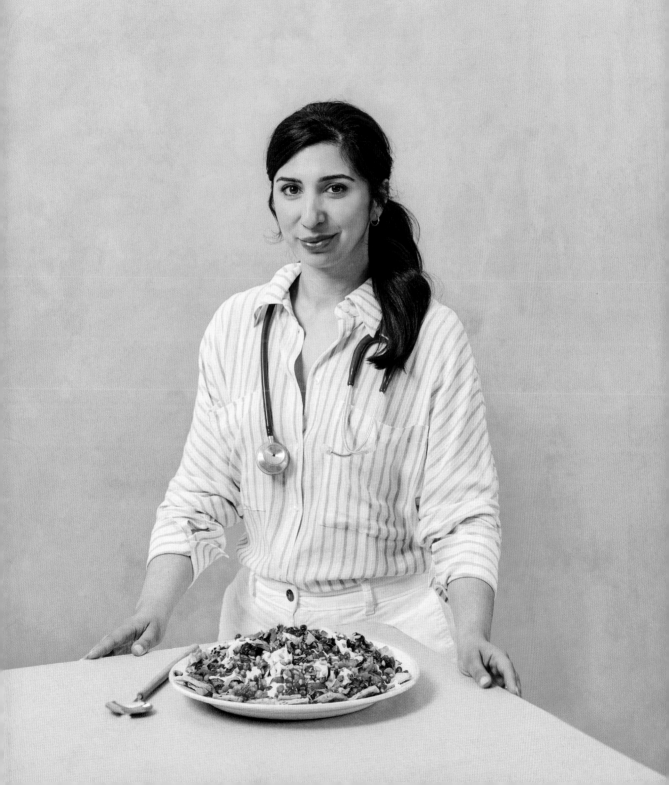

First published in Great Britain in 2023 by Yellow Kite
An imprint of Hodder & Stoughton
An Hachette UK company

1

A CIP catalogue record for this title is available from the British Library

Hardback 978 1 399 70629 2
eBook 978 1 399 70630 8

Editorial Director: Nicky Ross
Project Editor: Isabel Gonzalez-Prendergast
Assistant Editor: Olivia Nightingall
Art Direction & Design: Studio Nic&Lou
Photography: Steven Joyce
Food Stylist: Lizzie Harris
Props Stylist: Max Robinson
Production Manager: Claudette Morris

Colour origination by by Alta Image London
Printed and bound in in Germany by Mohn Media GmbH

Hodder & Stoughton policy is to use papers that are natural, renewable and recyclable products
and made from wood grown in sustainable forests. The logging and manufacturing processes are
expected to conform to the environmental regulations of the country of origin.

Yellow Kite
Hodder & Stoughton Ltd
Carmelite House
50 Victoria Embankment
London
EC4Y 0DZ
www.yellowkitebooks.co.uk